© *Copyright 20.*

The content contained within this book may not be reproduced, duplicated or transmitted without direct written permission from the author or the publisher.

Under no circumstances will any blame or legal responsibility be held against the publisher, or author, for any damages, reparation, or monetary loss due to the information contained within this book. Either directly or indirectly.

Legal Notice:

This book is copyright protected. This book is only for personal use. You cannot amend, distribute, sell, use, quote or paraphrase any part, or the content within this book, without the consent of the author or publisher.

Disclaimer Notice:

Please note the information contained within this document is for educational and entertainment purposes only. All effort has been executed to present accurate, up to date, and reliable, complete information. No warranties of any kind are declared or implied. Readers acknowledge that the author is not engaging in the rendering of legal, financial, medical or professional advice. The content within this book has been derived from various sources. Please consult a licensed professional before attempting any techniques outlined in this book.

By reading this document, the reader agrees that under no circumstances is the author responsible for any losses, direct or indirect, which are incurred as a result of the use of information contained within this document, including, but not limited to, — errors, omissions, or inaccuracies.

Table of Contents

Table of Contents 4

*License Notes****Errore. Il segnalibro non è definito.***

*Table of Contents****Errore. Il segnalibro non è definito.***

Introduction 10

    Sesame Salmon 11

    Basil & Parmesan Steaks 13

    Bell Pepper and Rice Soup 15

    Pegan Pancetta 17

    Oriental Inspired Rice Noodles and Stew Meat. 19

    Pegan Friendly Steak and Shrimp for Two 21

    Protein Stir Fry 23

    Grass-fed Burger Stew 25

    Flank Steak with Salad and a Homemade Vinaigrette 27

    Chicken Fajita Salad 29

    Pegan Spinach & Honey Turkey Pita 32

    Pegan Friendly Leek and Herb Gravy 34

    Pegan Cold Busting Soup 36

Cauliflower Steaks with Walnuts and Pomegranate 38

Pegan BBQ Chicken Pizza 40

Pegan Pizza Crust 42

Pegan Friendly Meatless Taco Meat 45

Pegan Veggie Stew 48

Pegan Cauliflower Rice with Baked Sesame Cod 51

Coconut Sesame Rice Noodles & Leek Casserole 54

Lunch .... **Errore. Il segnalibro non è definito.**

Rosemary Watermelon & Cucumber Salad 57

Pegan Cauliflower Gnocchi in a Creamy Sauce 60

Sweet Potato Gnocchi in an Herbed Dairy-Free Sauce 63

Jalapeno Mango Salad 66

Toasted Coconut and Walnut Zoodle Salad with Baked Chicken Tenders 69

Pegan Quinoa Salad and Baked Tuna 72

Cauli-Bites 75

Crispy Baked Chicken with Sweet Potato & Broccoli Tots 78

Mexican Sweet Tater Tots with Coconut-Cinnamon Pork Chops 80

Easy Grilled Veggie Turkey Sliders 82

Creamy Dairy-Free Veggie Soup 84

Roasted Veggies with Easy Homemade Tahini Sauce 86

Zoodle Noodle Salad with Easy Basil Dressing .. 89

Pegan Friendly Apple Crisps 92

G.F. Chocolate and Peanut Butter No-Bake Granola Bites 94

Vanilla Bean and Strawberry Dessert 96

Pegan Nutella 99

Pegan Friendly Cheesecake Bites in Caramel Sauce 101

Cool Mint Coconut Chia Pudding 104

Pegan Marshmallow Mint Brownies 107

Pegan Peanut Butter Brownies 110

Pegan Peanut Butter & Marshmallow Mint Brownies 113

Pagan Friendly Chocolate Loaf 116

Raspberry Frosting 119

Breakfast 121

Apple Pie Pegan Pancakes 122

Pegan Veggie Frittata 124
Eggs in Acorn Squash 126
Collard & Tomato Omelet 128
Herbed Mushrooms, Avocado and Eggs in a Bell Pepper 131
AM Smoothie 134
Easy Dairy-Free Latte 136

Author's Afterthoughts 138

Thanks ever so much to each of my cherished readers for investing the time to read this book! 138

About the Author 140

The Pegan Diet

50+ Pegan Diet Recipes. Easy Recipes for Healthy Weight Loss

BY

D.Robert Marshall

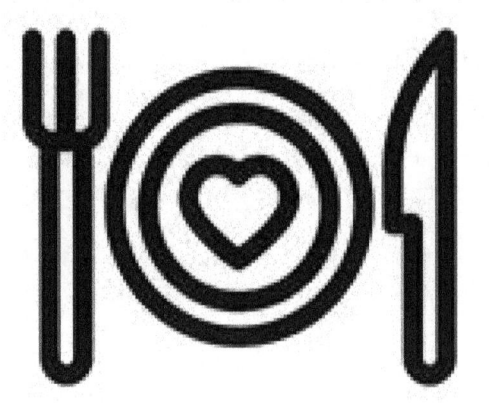

Copyright 2021 - D.Robert Marshall

Introduction

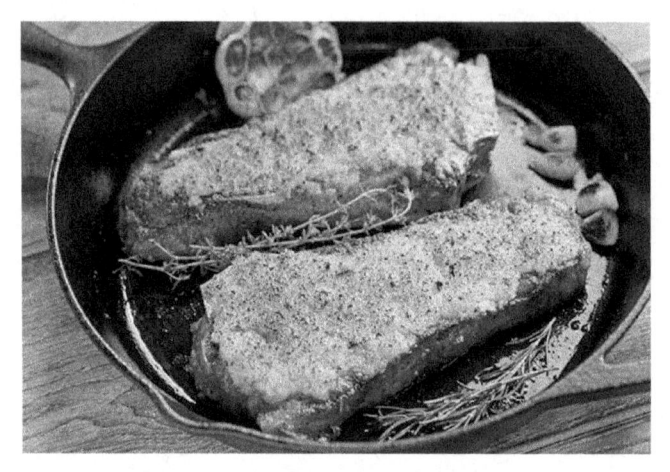

Need guidance in your Pegan diet? Need some new meal plans and ideas?

All recipes where devised within dietary guidelines; but, realize that by combining diverse diets, a variety of individual dietary needs are created. We have tried to formulate meal plans to accommodate this diversity or to be easily tailored to your specific wants and needs.

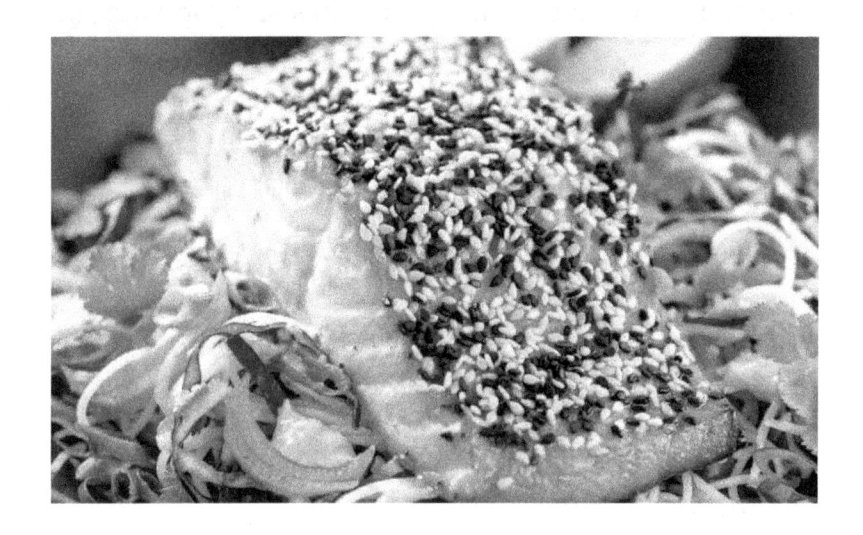

Sesame Salmon

Wild-caught, fresh fish is ok in moderation.

Makes: 2 servings.

Ingredients:

- 2 filets fresh wild-caught salmon
- ½ Tbsp brown sugar
- 1 stick butter
- 2 diced basil leaves

Directions:

In a skillet over medium-high heat melt butter into brown sugar.

Using a fork, poke holes into the flesh then lay fillets skin side down. Spoon butter over the fillets, focusing on drizzling it into the holes.

Cook 1-3 minutes per side, transfer to plates and top with diced basil.

Amount per Serving:

- *Total Fat 51.3g 66%*
- *Saturated Fat 29.8g 149%*
- *Cholesterol 161mg 54%*
- *Sodium 365mg 16%*
- *Total Carbohydrate 2.3g 1%*
- *Dietary Fiber 0g 0%*
- *Total Sugars 2.2g*
- *Protein 17.8g*
- *Vitamin D 32mcg 158%*
- *Calcium 48mg 4%*
- *Iron 1mg 3%*
- *Potassium 360mg*

Basil & Parmesan Steaks

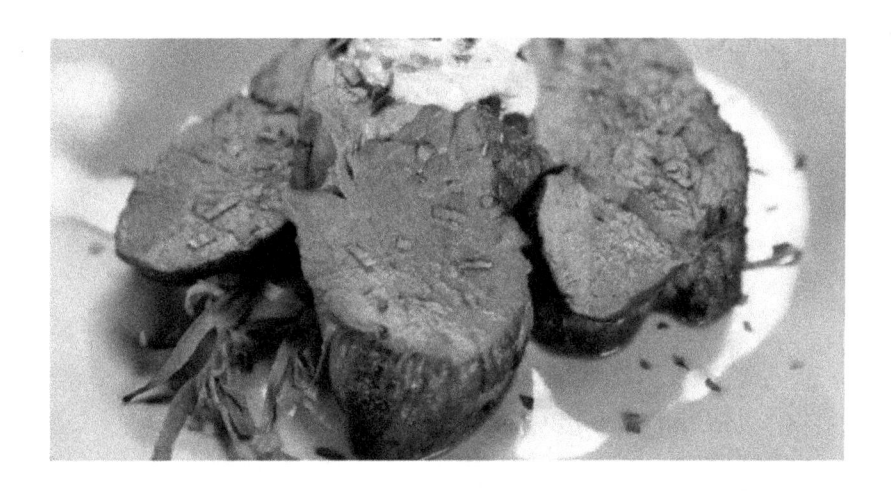

Red meats are great sources of vitamin B12!

Makes: 2 servings.

Ingredients:

- ½ tablespoon olive oil
- 2 cups of lean strips of steaks
- ½ tablespoon pine nuts
- ½ cup diced mushrooms
- ½ tablespoons diced parsley
- ½ tablespoon diced oregano

Directions:

In a hot skillet cook steak strips over olive oil approx. 1 minute and transfer to plates.

Sauté pine nuts and mushroom 30-45 seconds and spoon over steak strips before topping with parsley and oregano.

Amount per Serving:

- Calories 191
- % Daily Value*
- Total Fat 5.9g 8%
- Saturated Fat 1.6g 8%
- Cholesterol 77mg 26%
- Sodium 40mg 2%
- Total Carbohydrate 1.7g 1%
- Dietary Fiber 0.8g 3%
- Total Sugars 0.4g
- Protein 31.7g
- Vitamin D 63mcg 315%
- Calcium 23mg 2%
- Iron 4mg 22%
- Potassium 377mg 8

Bell Pepper and Rice Soup

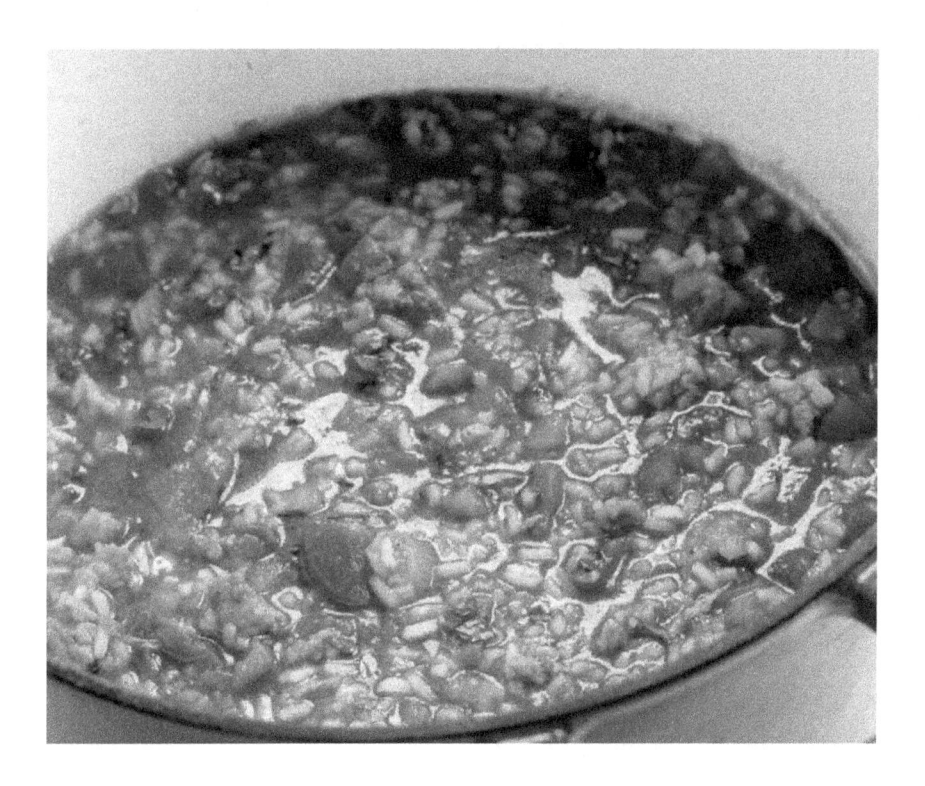

Delicious!

Makes: 1 serving.

Ingredients:

- 3 cups organic vegetable broth
- ½ cup basmati rice
- 1 red bell pepper, julienned
- ½ Tbsp diced thyme
- 1/3 teaspoon black pepper
- 2 oz leftover ground beef or hamburger crumble (optional)

Directions:

In a pot bring broth, rice kernels, julienned bell pepper, thyme, pepper, and ground beef to a boil.

Reduce heat, cover, and let simmer 15-20 minutes.

With hamburger-

Amount per Serving:

- *Calories 505*
- *% Daily Value**
- *Total Fat 4.5g 6%*
- *Saturated Fat 1.5g 8%*
- *Cholesterol 51mg 17%*
- *Sodium 596mg 26%*
- *Total Carbohydrate 85.8g 31%*
- *Dietary Fiber 3.3g 12%*
- *Total Sugars 8.1g*
- *Protein 27.1g*
- *Vitamin D 0mcg 0%*
- *Calcium 82mg 6%*
- *Iron 14mg 78%*
- *Potassium 570mg 12*

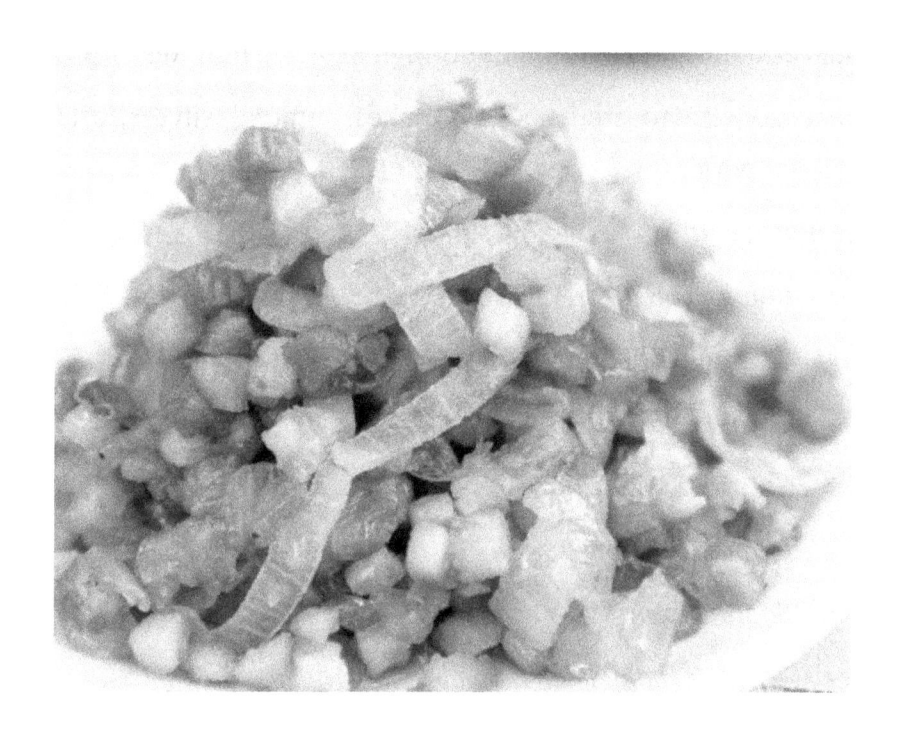

Pegan Pancetta

Great over rice or in a wrap!

Makes: 1 9x9 pan.

Ingredients:

- 1 cup of pancetta
- ½ cup toasted coconut flakes
- ½ cup toasted almond slivers
- ¾ cup multicolored bell peppers, diced
- Non-stick cooking spray

Directions:

Sauté pancetta in skillet over medium-high heat 1-2 minutes.

Mix pancetta with toasted coconut flakes, almond slivers, and diced bell peppers.

Amount per Serving:

- *Calories 68*
- *% Daily Value**
- *Total Fat 5.7g 7%*
- *Saturated Fat 1.8g 9%*
- *Cholesterol 2mg 1%*
- *Sodium 52mg 2%*
- *Total Carbohydrate 2.8g 1%*
- *Dietary Fiber 1.2g 4%*
- *Total Sugars 1g*
- *Protein 2.4g*
- *Vitamin D 0mcg 0%*
- *Calcium 14mg 1%*
- *Iron 1mg 5%*
- *Potassium 46mg 1%*

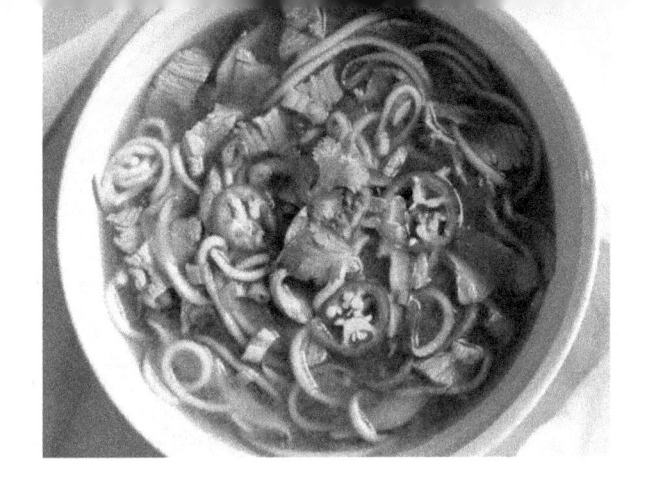

Oriental Inspired Rice Noodles and Stew Meat

Stews are great for small portions of meat and heavy on the veggies!

Makes: 4 servings.

Ingredients:

- 1 teaspoon sesame oil
- ¼ teaspoon chili oil or paste
- ½ teaspoon ginger paste
- 1 teaspoon sweet paprika
- 1-pound stew meat
- 2 cloves garlic, thinly sliced
- ½ cup matchstick carrots
- 1 fresh jalapeno peppers, diced
- 1 can organic diced tomatoes
- 1 onion, sliced
- 4 cups beef or vegetable broth
- 1 cup worth rice noodles
- ½ teaspoon diced oregano

Directions:

Brown stew meat and drain.

In crock pot combine sesame oil, chili oil or paste, ginger paste, sweet paprika, browned stew meat, ginger, matchstick carrots, jalapeno peppers, organic diced tomatoes, diced onion, and broth.

Let cook 30 minutes and add rice noodles and diced oregano.

Amount per Serving:

- *Calories 421*
- *% Daily Value**
- *Total Fat 18g 23%*
- *Saturated Fat 6.4g 32%*
- *Cholesterol 120mg 40%*
- *Sodium 959mg 42%*
- *Total Carbohydrate 20.3g 7%*
- *Dietary Fiber 2.7g 10%*
- *Total Sugars 5.1g*
- *Protein 41.9g*
- *Vitamin D 0mcg 0%*
- *Calcium 53mg 4%*
- *Iron 5mg 30%*
- *Potassium 827mg 18%*

Pegan Friendly Steak and Shrimp for Two

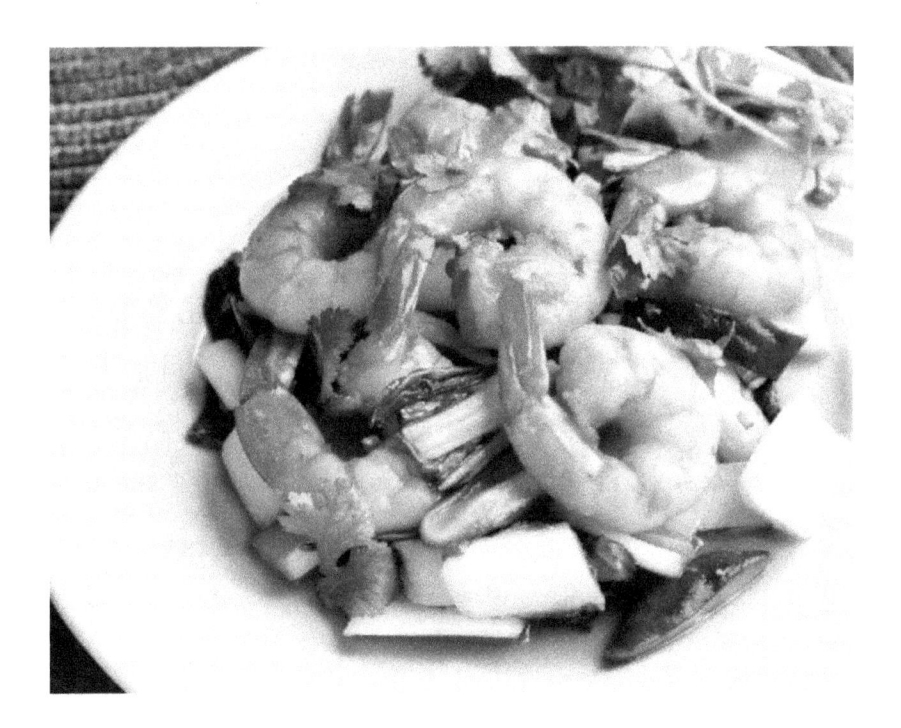

The trick here is to limit portion size.

Makes: 2 servings.

Ingredients:

- 2 3 - oz. sirloin steaks
- 8 medium shrimp
- 2 tablespoon butter or ghee
- 2/3 tablespoon white wine
- 1/3 teaspoon chicken granules
- 1 teaspoon paprika
- ½ teaspoon pepper

- 2 diced scallions
- 1 teaspoon Worcestershire sauce
- ½ teaspoon chili powder
- 1 teaspoon diced parsley
- 1/3 cup sliced mushrooms
- ¼ cup pine nuts (optional)

Directions:

In a plastic bag combine shrimp, butter or ghee, white wine, chicken granules, parsley, paprika, pepper. Marinate in fridge 30 minutes.

Mix together Worcestershire sauce, chili powder, parsley, sliced mushrooms, then cook steak 4-5 minutes per side.

Transfer done steaks to a plate and top with mushroom mix and pine nuts.

Cook shrimp 1-2 minutes, transfer to plate, and serve.

Protein Stir Fry

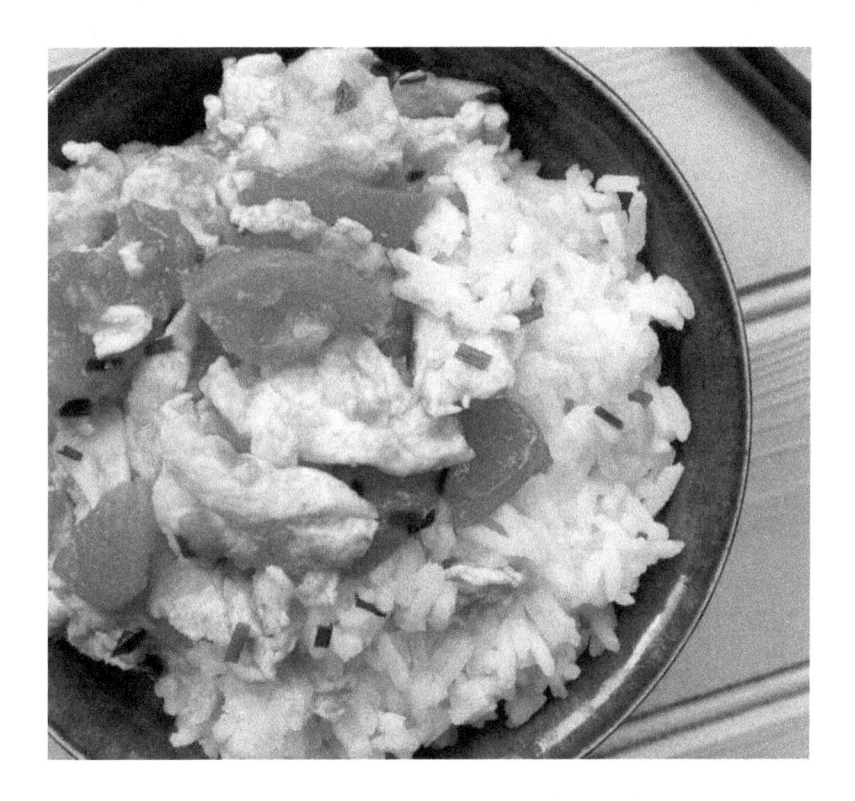

Great for breakfast or dinner!

Makes: 4 servings.

Ingredients:

- Coconut or avocado oil
- 6-7 eggs, beaten
- 4 plum tomatoes, sliced into wedges
- 2 scallions, thinly sliced
- 1 teaspoon turmeric
- Favorite herbs

Directions:

Scramble eggs and stir in sliced tomatoes, sliced scallions, turmeric and diced herbs.

Amount per Serving:

- Calories 478
- % Daily Value*
- Total Fat 40g 51%
- Saturated Fat 31.5g 157%
- Cholesterol 246mg 82%
- Sodium 130mg 6%
- Total Carbohydrate 22.8g 8%
- Dietary Fiber 10.6g 38%
- Total Sugars 11.8g
- Protein 13.3g
- Vitamin D 23mcg 116%
- Calcium 59mg 5%
- Iron 16mg 89%
- Potassium 727mg

Grass-fed Burger Stew

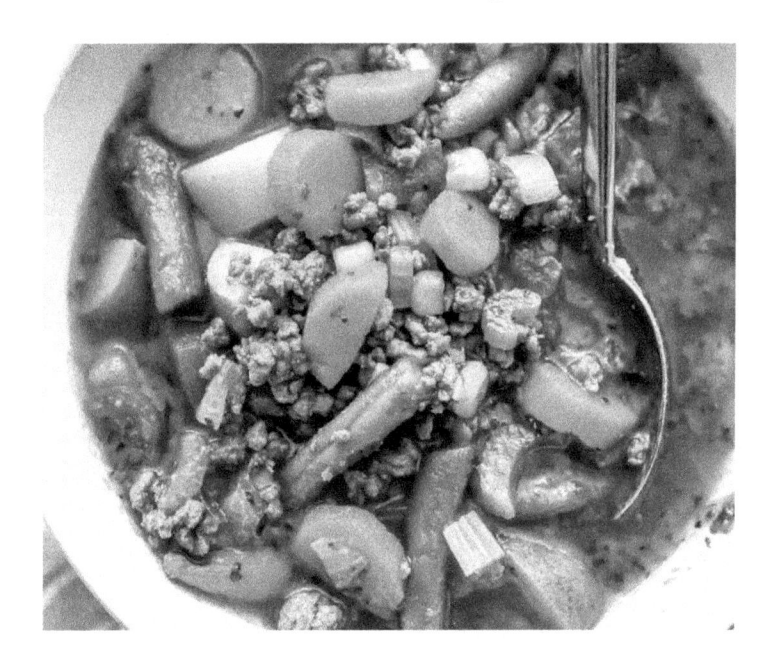

75% of this diet is dedicated to veggies, making in perfect for stews!

Makes: 4 servings.

Ingredients:

- ½ cup diced onions
- 1 teaspoon minced garlic
- 1.2 teaspoon pepper
- ½-pound grass-fed ground beef, browned and drained
- 4 cups brussel sprouts
- ½ cup matchstick carrots
- ½ cup peas or edamame
- 4 cups organic vegetable broth

Directions:

In crockpot add onions, garlic, pepper, browned beef, brussel sprouts, matchstick carrots, peas or edamame, vegetable broth.

Cook on high heat 30-45 minutes.

Amount per Serving:

- Calories 199
- % Daily Value*
- Total Fat 7.3g 9%
- Saturated Fat 2.8g 14%
- Cholesterol 38mg 13%
- Sodium 825mg 36%
- Total Carbohydrate 13.3g 5%
- Dietary Fiber 4.6g 16%
- Total Sugars 4.3g
- Protein 20.6g
- Vitamin D 0mcg 0%
- Calcium 60mg 5%
- Iron 3mg 18%
- Potassium 620mg 13%

Flank Steak with Salad and a Homemade Vinaigrette

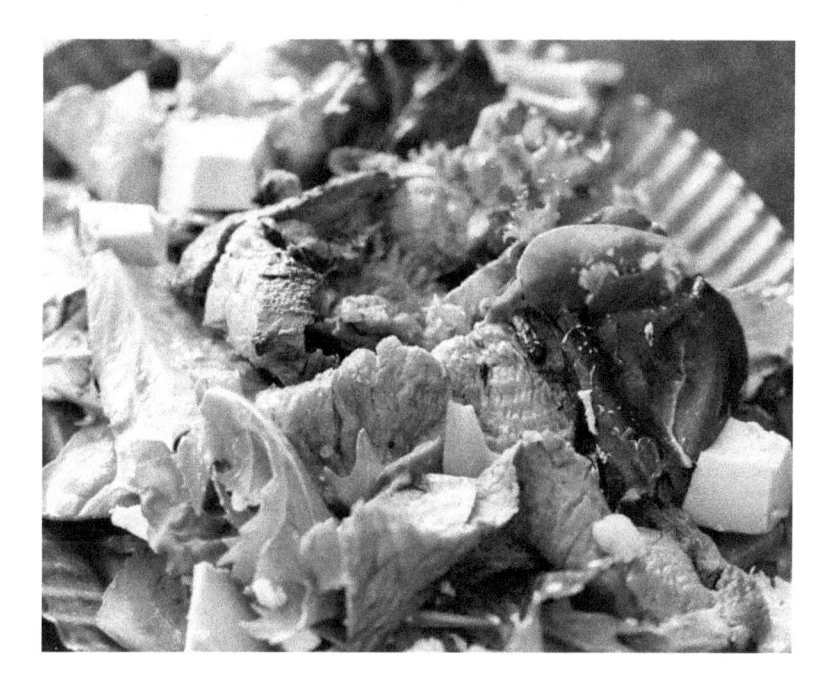

If desired, add shredded cheese and chopped walnuts to salad.

Makes: 2 servings

Ingredients:

- 2/3 cup extra-virgin olive oil
- ¼ teaspoon red wine vinegar
- ¼ cup chopped herbs
- 1 clove garlic, minced
- 3 cups chopped lettuce
- 2 chopped plum tomatoes
- 2 3 oz. Flank steak
- 1 teaspoon steak seasoning

Directions:

Mix together olive oil, red wine vinegar, chopped herbs, minced garlic; cover and sit in refrigerator.

Combine lettuce and tomatoes; chill.

Bring steaks to room temp, season and grill steaks 4-5 minutes per side.

Amount per Serving:

- *Calories 1210*
- *% Daily Value**
- *Total Fat 94g 121%*
- *Saturated Fat 20.7g 103%*
- *Cholesterol 176mg 59%*
- *Sodium 181mg 8%*
- *Total Carbohydrate 3g 1%*
- *Dietary Fiber 1.7g 6%*
- *Total Sugars 0.1g*
- *Protein 89.7g*
- *Vitamin D 0mcg 0%*
- *Calcium 139mg 11%*
- *Iron 8mg 43%*
- *Potassium 1232mg 26%*

Chicken Fajita Salad

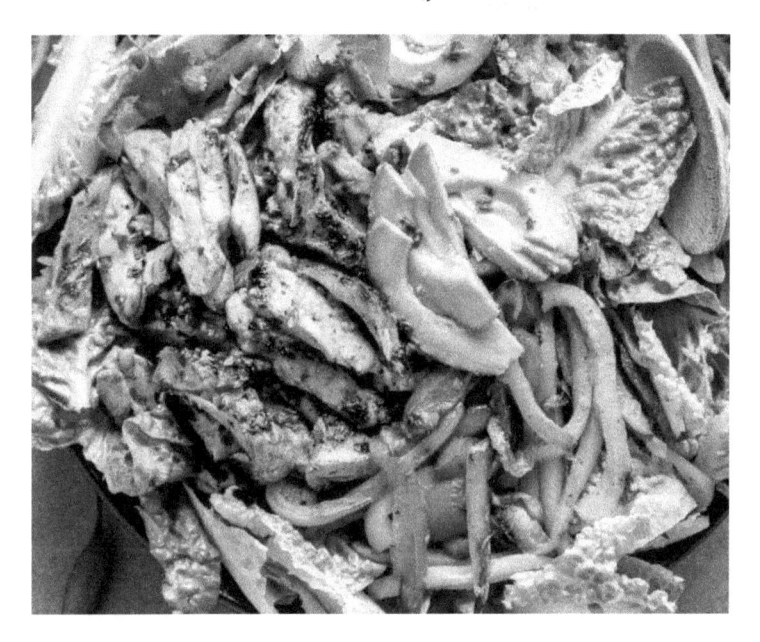

Ground chicken works too!

Makes: 2 servings.

Ingredients:

- ½ pound stir fry chicken strips
- 1 bell pepper, julienned
- 4 cups shredded lettuce
- 2-3 diced tomatoes
- 1 can organic black beans, washed
- ½ tablespoon lime juice
- 1 tablespoons chili powder
- 1 teaspoon ground cumin
- 1 teaspoon ground coriander

- 1 teaspoon brown sugar
- ¼ teaspoon cayenne pepper
- 4-5 gluten free pita chips

Directions:

In a plastic bag combine chicken strips, lime juice, chili powder, ground cumin, coriander, brown sugar, cayenne pepper.

Combine lettuce, tomatoes, and black beans then let chill in refrigerator.

Sauté chicken and peppers in skillet over olive oil 1-2 minutes; add to lettuce, tomatoes, and black beans and toss.

mount per serving

Amount per Serving:

- *Calories 313*
- *% Daily Value**
- *Total Fat 7.1g 9%*
- *Saturated Fat 0.4g 2%*
- *Cholesterol 65mg 22%*
- *Sodium 332mg 14%*
- *Total Carbohydrate 34g 12%*
- *Dietary Fiber 6.2g 22%*
- *Total Sugars 11.4g*
- *Protein 32g*
- *Vitamin D 0mcg 0%*

- *Calcium 79mg 6%*
- *Iron 6mg 35%*
- *Potassium 815mg 17%*

Pegan Spinach & Honey Turkey Pita

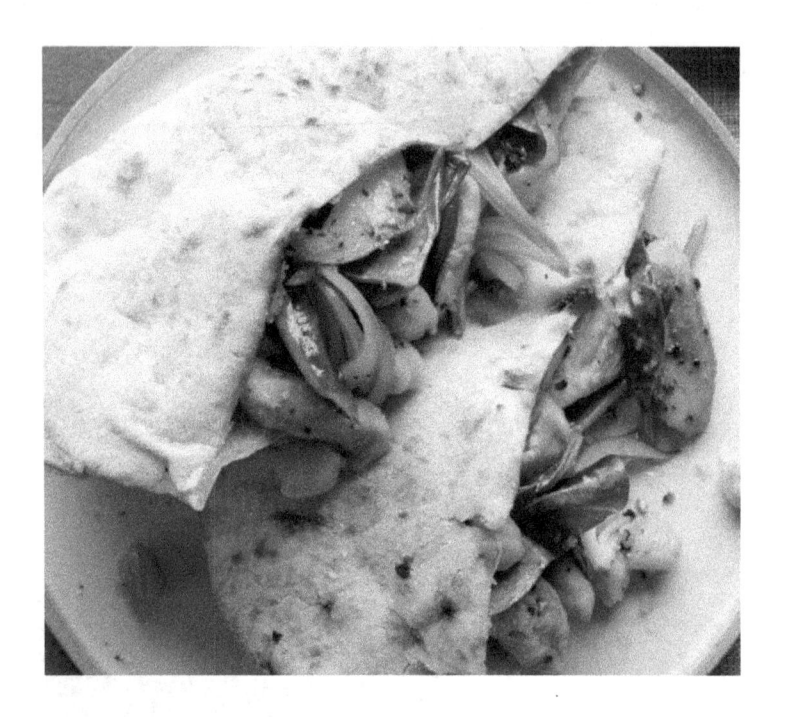

Also, great as a wrap!

Makes: 2 servings.

Ingredients:

- 2 4-inch whole wheat pitas
- 2 cups leftover shredded turkey
- ½ cup baby spinach leaves
- 1/3 cup bell pepper, diced
- 2 teaspoons organic honey
- 1 teaspoon walnuts

Directions:

In a small bowl mix together shredded turkey, diced bell peppers, honey, and walnuts.

Fill each pita shell with half of baby spinach leaves then fill with half of turkey mixture.

Amount per Serving:

- *Calories 235*
- *% Daily Value**
- *Total Fat 3.1g 4%*
- *Saturated Fat 0.4g 2%*
- *Cholesterol 11mg 4%*
- *Sodium 618mg 27%*
- *Total Carbohydrate 43.8g 16%*
- *Dietary Fiber 5.3g 19%*
- *Total Sugars 7.5g*
- *Protein 11.8g*
- *Vitamin D 0mcg 0%*
- *Calcium 22mg 2%*
- *Iron 3mg 14%*
- *Potassium 261mg 6%*

Pegan Friendly Leek and Herb Gravy

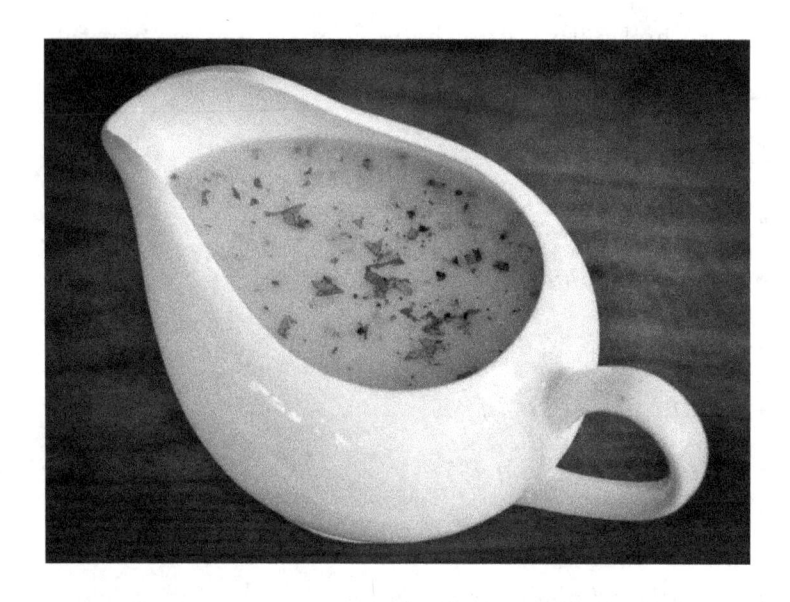

Only use the white and pale green parts of the leeks!

Makes: 8 servings.

Ingredients:

- 2/3 cup diced leek
- 1 cup dry white wine
- 2 cups chicken stock or water
- ¼ cup all-purpose gluten free rice flour blend
- 1 teaspoon finely diced Italian oregano
- 1 teaspoon finely diced lemon thyme
- 1 teaspoon finely diced rosemary

Directions:

To skillet add flour, stirring frequently, and toast 1 minute (will become fragrant and a light brown).

Whisk in stock/water, wine, and diced leeks.

Bring to a boil, cover, reduce heat and simmer 25-30 minutes or until reduced by half. Stir occasionally.

Stir in diced oregano, thyme, and rosemary.

Amount per Serving:

- Calories 36
- % Daily Value*
- Total Fat 0.2g 0%
- Saturated Fat 0.1g 0%
- Cholesterol 0mg 0%
- Sodium 198mg 9%
- Total Carbohydrate 3.1g 1%
- Dietary Fiber 0.3g 1%
- Total Sugars 0.7g
- Protein 0.4g
- Vitamin D 0mcg 0%
- Calcium 18mg 1%
- Iron 1mg 3%
- Potassium 52mg 1%

Pegan Cold Busting Soup

For bronchial help add rosemary!

Makes: 2-3 servings.

Ingredients:

- 1 tablespoon Beau Monde seasoning
- 1 bouquet of herbs*
- 1/3 cup matchstick carrots
- 1 cup shiitake mushrooms, sliced
- 1-inch fresh ginger, diced OR 1 teaspoon ground ginger
- 1-inch fresh turmeric, diced OR 1 teaspoon of ground turmeric
- ½ tsp peppercorns
- 4 cups shredded chicken meat
- 6-8 cups bone stock

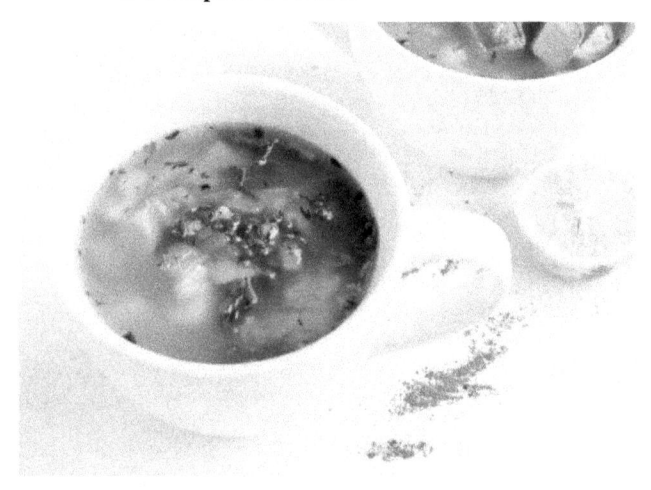

Directions:

In pot combine Beau Monde seasoning, herbs, matchstick carrots, ginger, turmeric, peppercorns, chicken, stock

Bring to a boil, cover, reduce heat and let simmer 10-15 minutes.

Bouquet of herb is a bunch of herbs tied together

mount per serving

Amount per Serving:

- *Calories 765*
- *% Daily Value**
- *Total Fat 21.1g 27%*
- *Saturated Fat 5.8g 29%*
- *Cholesterol 249mg 83%*
- *Sodium 877mg 38%*
- *Total Carbohydrate 13g 5%*
- *Dietary Fiber 2.3g 8%*
- *Total Sugars 3.5g*
- *Protein 124.5g*
- *Vitamin D 0mcg 0%*
- *Calcium 53mg 4%*
- *Iron 4mg 25%*
- *Potassium 812mg 17%*

Cauliflower Steaks with Walnuts and Pomegranate

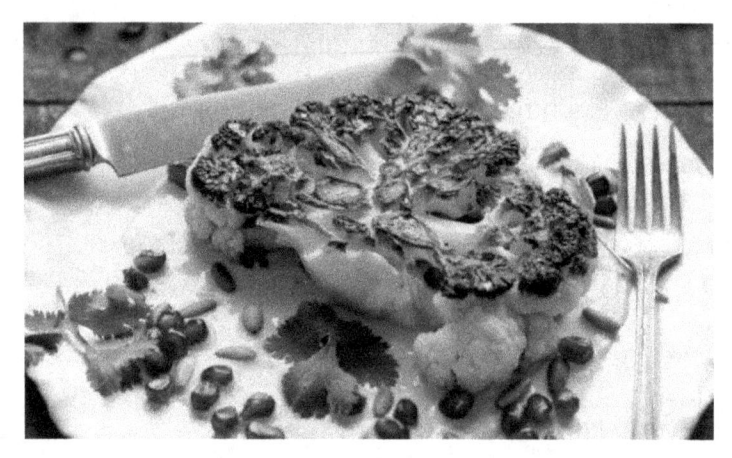

Also, great with raisins or cranberries! Pomegranates have many anti-inflammatory properties!

Makes: 4 servings.

Ingredients:

- 4 cauliflower steaks
- Olive oil for drizzling
- ¼ cup walnuts
- ¼ cup pomegranates
- 4 basil leaves, coarsely chopped
- Pumpkin or soy seeds (optional)

Directions:

Preheat oven to 350 and line baking tray with parchment paper.

Lay steaks on tray, drizzle with oil and sprinkle with walnuts and pomegranates. Bake 10-15 minutes.

Top with pieces of basil and seeds before serving!

Amount per Serving:

- *Calories 139*
- *% Daily Value**
- *Total Fat 8.6g 11%*
- *Saturated Fat 0.8g 4%*
- *Cholesterol 0mg 0%*
- *Sodium 53mg 2%*
- *Total Carbohydrate 13g 5%*
- *Dietary Fiber 4.7g 17%*
- *Total Sugars 4.1g*
- *Protein 6.4g*
- *Vitamin D 0mcg 0%*
- *Calcium 81mg 6%*
- *Iron 1mg 8%*
- *Potassium 571mg*

Pegan BBQ Chicken Pizza

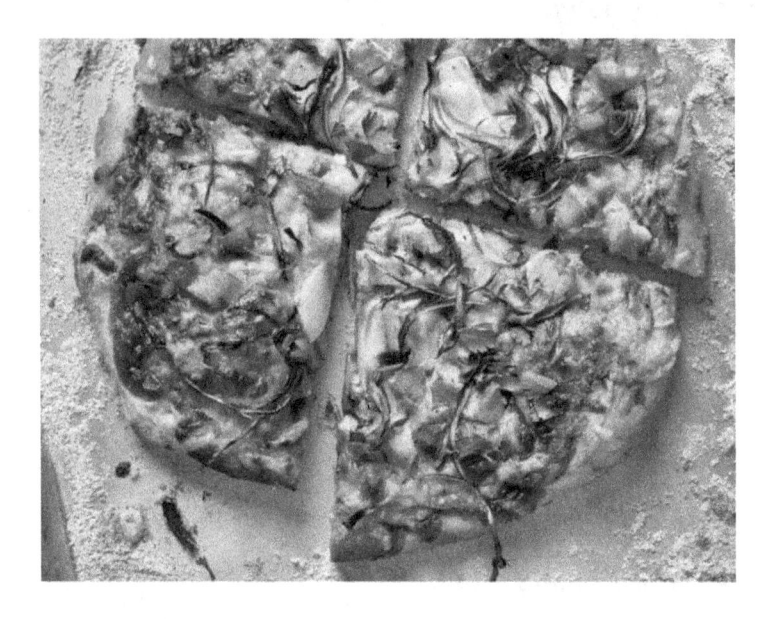

Enjoy the night out with family, friends, and pizza!

Makes: 1 12-14-inch crust, approx. 8 slices

Ingredients:

- 1 cup chicken breasts, shredded
- ¼ cup fav healthy BBQ sauce
- 1 cup mozzarella OR Italian blend shredded cheese
- 1 small onion sliced
- ¼ teaspoon Italian seasoning
- 1 paleo pizza crust* see recipe below

Directions:

Preheat oven to 350.

Make paleo pizza crust and spread on BBQ sauce.

Top with shredded chicken, cheese, onion, seasoning.

Cook 12-14 minutes.

Amount per Serving:

- Calories 48
- % Daily Value*
- Total Fat 2g 3%
- Saturated Fat 0.8g 4%
- Cholesterol 18mg 6%
- Sodium 44mg 2%
- Total Carbohydrate 1.2g 0%
- Dietary Fiber 0.2g 1%
- Total Sugars 0.6g
- Protein 6.2g
- Vitamin D 0mcg 0%
- Calcium 7mg 1%
- Iron 0mg 1%
- Potassium 57mg 1%

Pegan Pizza Crust

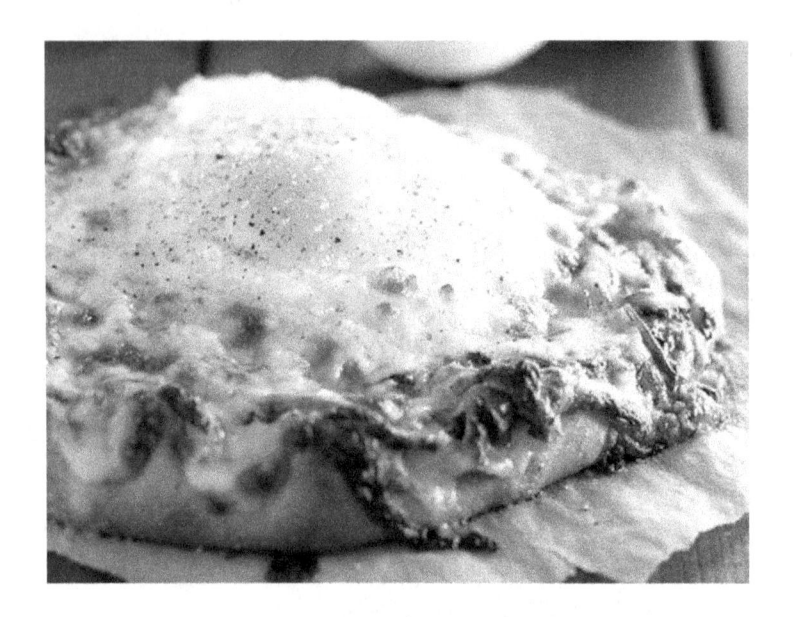

Great for all pizzas!

Makes: 1 12-14-inch pizza crust.

Ingredients:

- ¾ cup + 2 tablespoons tapioca flour
- 1/3 cup + 2 tablespoons coconut flour
- 1/3 teaspoon sea salt
- ½ cup olive oil
- ½ cup warm water
- 1 large egg

Directions:

Preheat oven to 450 and prepare pizza stone.

Mix together tapioca flour, coconut flour, and salt. Pour in olive oil and water. Add in egg and stir well.

Dough should be a little sticky, form into a ball and empty unto a hard surface sprinkled with tapioca flour. Knead 1-3 minutes or until it forms a non-sticky ball.

Transfer unto parchment parch and with a rolling pin dusted with tapioca powder roll out dough to a 12-14-inch crust. If needed dust rolling pin or pizza with more tapioca flour. However, stay mindful of how much is used as to much will make it dense.

Transfer rolled out dough to prepared pizza stone and bake 12-15 minutes.

Amount per Serving:

- Calories 173
- % Daily Value*
- Total Fat 13.7g 18%
- Saturated Fat 2.3g 11%
- Cholesterol 20mg 7%
- Sodium 86mg 4%
- Total Carbohydrate 13.1g 5%
- Dietary Fiber 2g 7%
- Total Sugars 0g
- Protein 1.4g
- Vitamin D 2mcg 10%
- Calcium 3mg 0%

- *Iron 0mg 1%*
- *Potassium 8mg 0%*

Pegan Friendly Meatless Taco Meat

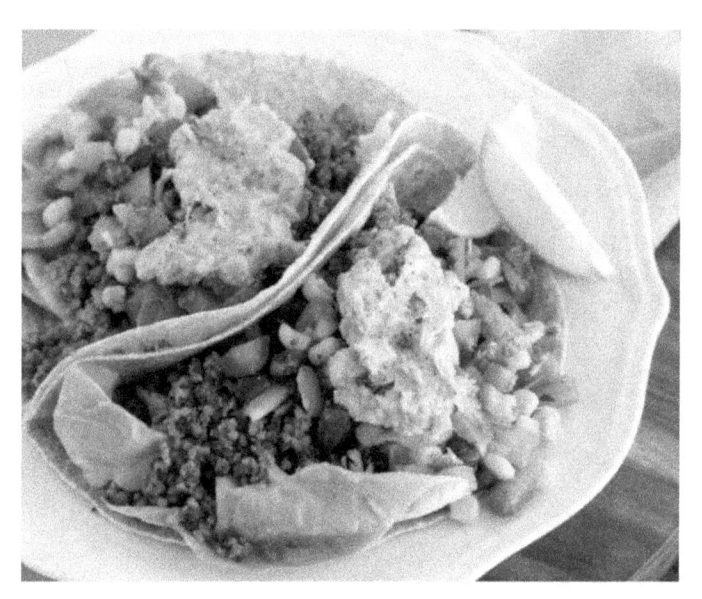

Great for stir-fry's too!

Makes: approx. 4-6 cups.

Ingredients:

Taco Meat

- ¾ cup +1 tablespoon chopped walnuts
- 1 cup cauliflower florets
- ½ cup sliced baby shitake or button mushrooms
- 2 teaspoons olive oil or avocado oil
- 2 tablespoons nutritional yeast

Taco Spice Mixture

- 1 ½ teaspoons chili powder
- 1 ½ teaspoons of smoked paprika
- ½ teaspoon garlic powder
- 1 teaspoon cumin
- ½ teaspoons onion powder
- 1 teaspoon oregano
- ¼ teaspoon pepper
- 1 tablespoon coconut sugar
- ½ tablespoon organic honey

Directions:

Preheat 350

Toast walnuts by spreading on baking tray and cooking about 10 minutes.

Turn oven up to 400

Transfer to a bowl then place cauliflower, sliced mushrooms to the sheet. Drizzle with oil and roast 18-22 minutes or until edges of cauliflower starts to turn at edges.

Meanwhile mix together chili powder, smoked paprika, garlic powder, cumin, onion powder, pepper, oregano, coconut sugar, organic honey.

Blend together walnuts, nutritional yeast, and spice mix together and 1 teaspoon at a time mix into meat. Once desired taste is achieved store remaining mix in an airtight container in the refrigerator.

Make ahead will keep 5 days in fridge or 1 month in freezer!

Amount per Serving:

- Calories 176
- % Daily Value*
- Total Fat 13.5g 17%
- Saturated Fat 1g 5%
- Cholesterol 0mg 0%
- Sodium 18mg 1%
- Total Carbohydrate 10.7g 4%
- Dietary Fiber 3.6g 13%
- Total Sugars 5.2g
- Protein 7.2g
- Vitamin D 1mcg 3%
- Calcium 33mg 3%
- Iron 2mg 12%
- Potassium 313mg 7%

Pegan Veggie Stew

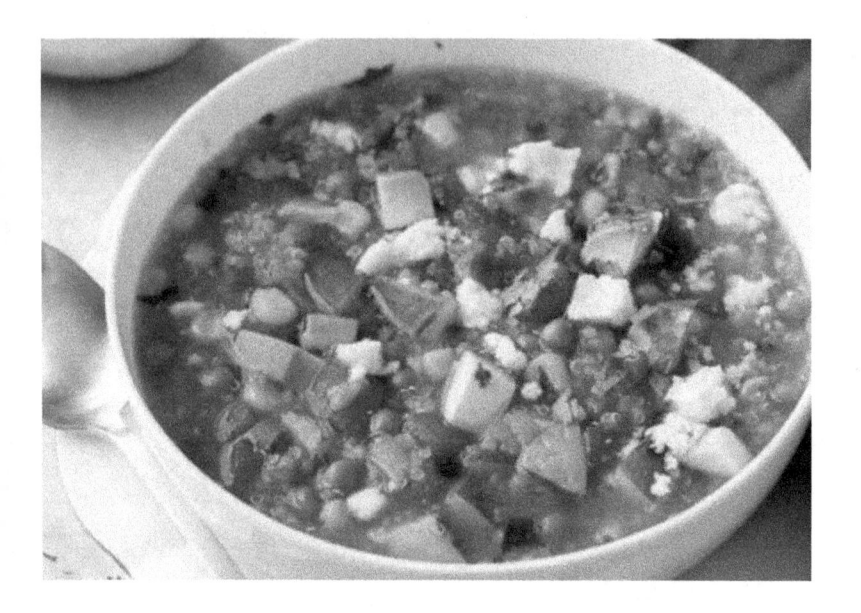

For added texture add in rice noodles!

Makes: 4 servings.

Ingredients:

- 1 tablespoon olive oil or coconut oil
- 1 tsp cayenne powder
- 1/3 cup onion, diced
- 1 clove garlic thinly sliced
- 1/3 cup diced red bell pepper
- 1 large eggplant, cubed
- 2 zucchinis, sliced
- ¼ cup mushrooms, diced
- 2/3 tablespoon organic tomato paste

- 1 large can petite diced no-salt added tomatoes
- 2 tbs fresh thyme
- 2 cups water, chicken stock, or veggie stock
- ¼ c fresh basil
- ¼ c fresh parsley

Directions:

In a Dutch oven brought to medium heat add olive oil, cayenne powder, diced onions, garlic slices, diced red bell peppers. Sauté 3-5 minutes.

Add in eggplant cubes and zucchini slices let meld 1 minute.

Stir in tomato paste, petite diced tomatoes, a liquid. Bring to boil, cover, reduce heat and simmer 20 minutes.

Remove from heat and stir in all herbs.

Amount per Serving:

- Calories 92
- % Daily Value*
- Total Fat 4.2g 5%
- Saturated Fat 0.6g 3%
- Cholesterol 0mg 0%
- Sodium 23mg 1%
- Total Carbohydrate 13.9g 5%
- Dietary Fiber 6.4g 23%
- Total Sugars 6.6g

- *Protein 3.2g*
- *Vitamin D 16mcg 79%*
- *Calcium 68mg 5%*
- *Iron 3mg 16%*
- *Potassium 643mg 14%*

Pegan Cauliflower Rice with Baked Sesame Cod

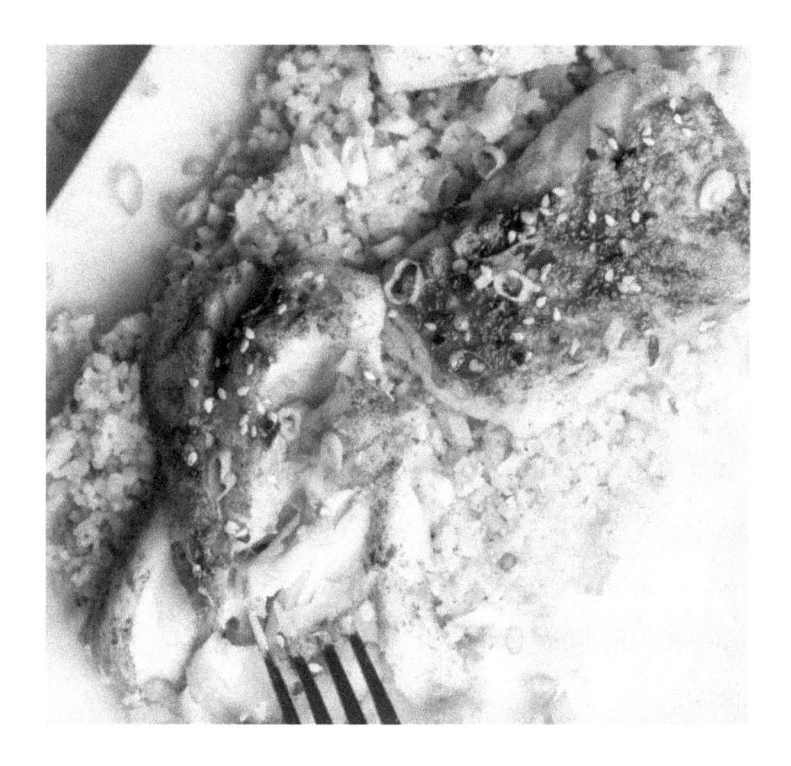

Great with red fish too!

Makes: 4 servings.

Ingredients:

- 4 cups cauliflower rice
- 2 teaspoons olive oil
- 1 tablespoon butter or ghee
- 2 tablespoons onion, chopped
- 1 teaspoon garlic, minced
- 2/3 teaspoon lemon peel
- 1 teaspoon picante seasoning

- 2/3 teaspoon black pepper
- 2 tablespoons pinenuts
- ¼ cup parsley, chopped
- ¼ cup Italian oregano, diced
- 4 filets of cod
- 3 packet, or 3 cups, chicken stock

Directions:

Preheat oven to 350 and prepare 13x13 dish.

Place filets in dish and pour liquid around them. Bake 30 minutes.

To skillet warmed over medium-high heat add olive oil, butter, onion, garlic sauté 3-5 minutes then stir in cauliflower.

Sprinkle over cauliflower picante seasoning, black pepper.

Divide amongst four plates and top each with pinenuts, parsley, Italian oregano

Servings: 4

Amount per Serving:

- *Calories 90*
- *% Daily Value**
- *Total Fat 7.6g 10%*
- *Saturated Fat 2.8g 14%*
- *Cholesterol 8mg 3%*
- *Sodium 620mg 27%*
- *Total Carbohydrate 4.2g 2%*

- *Dietary Fiber 1.4g 5%*
- *Total Sugars 1.4g*
- *Protein 1.8g*
- *Vitamin D 2mcg 10%*
- *Calcium 26mg 2%*
- *Iron 1mg 3%*
- *Potassium 48mg 1%*

-Coconut Sesame Rice Noodles & Leek Casserole

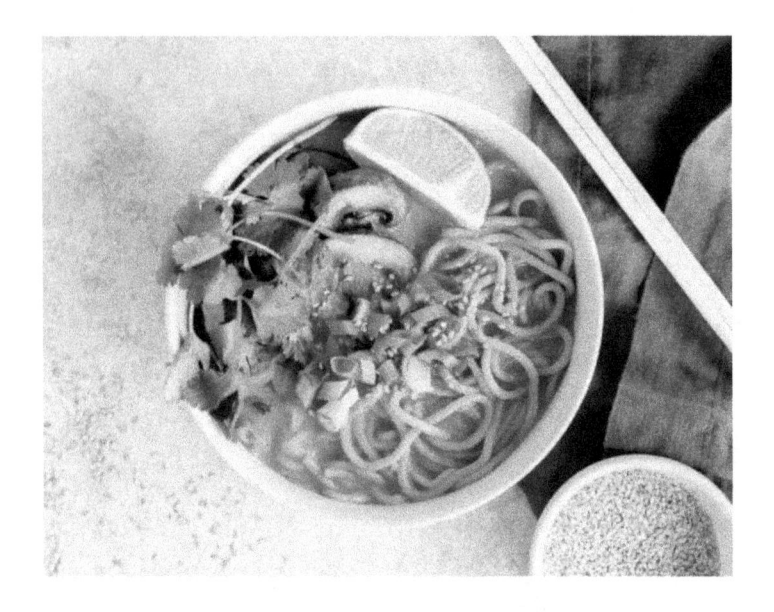

For added Protein add chickpeas or black beans.

Makes: 4 servings.

Ingredients:

- 1 teaspoon sesame oil
- 1 ½ tablespoon coconut oil
- 2 leeks, washed and sliced
- ½ teaspoon garlic, minced
- 1/3 cup mirepoix
- 1 cup potatoes, cubed
- 1 cup edamame
- 1 cup asparagus spears
- 1 can organic crushed or stewed tomatoes

- 1 ¼ cup + 1 tablespoon beef or veggie stock (water works too)
- ½ cup worth rice noodles, uncooked

Directions:

In Dutch oven add coconut oil, sliced leeks, minced garlic, mirepoix and sauté 2-3 minutes. Add in cubed potatoes, edamame, asparagus s-pears, tomatoes, stock or water, uncooked rice noodles. Stir well.

Bring to a boil, cover, reduce heat, let simmer 20-25

Servings: 4

Amount per Serving:

- *Calories 262*
- *% Daily Value**
- *Total Fat 11.1g 14%*
- *Saturated Fat 5.2g 26%*
- *Cholesterol 0mg 0%*
- *Sodium 275mg 12%*
- *Total Carbohydrate 31.7g 12%*
- *Dietary Fiber 5.6g 20%*
- *Total Sugars 2.8g*
- *Protein 11.6g*
- *Vitamin D 0mcg 0%*
- *Calcium 171mg 13%*

- *Iron 4mg 24%*
- *Potassium 741mg 16%*

Rosemary Watermelon & Cucumber Salad

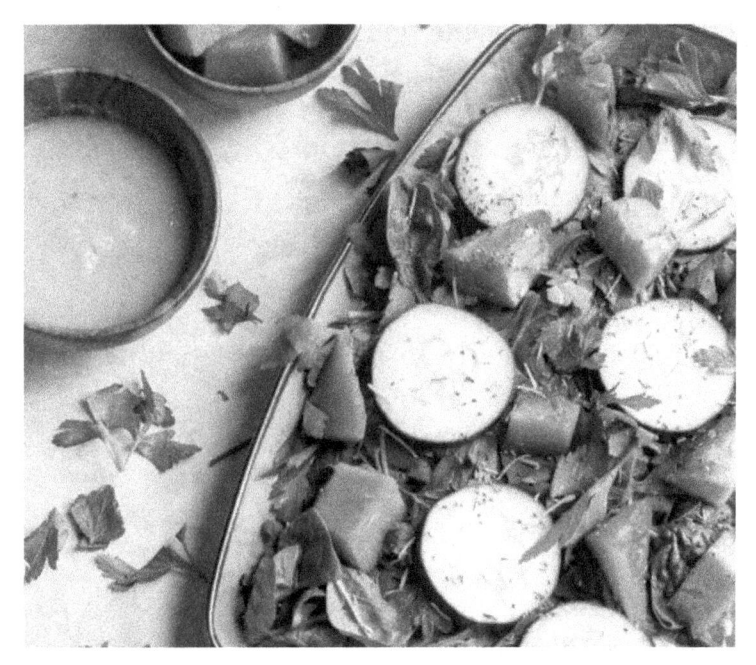

Serve with low-carb pita chips!

Makes: 4-6 servings.

Ingredients:

- 1 can of garbanzo beans drained and washed (chickpeas)
- 4 cups chunked watermelon
- 1 seedless cucumber, sliced
- 1 cup olive oil
- ½ teaspoon of red or white wine vinegar
- ½ tablespoon rosemary, diced
- ½ tablespoon Italian oregano, diced
- ½ tablespoon parsley, diced

- 2 diced scallions

Directions:

Mix together olive oil, wine vinegar, diced rosemary, diced oregano, diced parsley, diced scallions. Cover and chill.

In a large bowl mix together drained and washed garbanzo beans, watermelon chunks, cucumber slices.

Pour vinaigrette over salad, toss, serve!

Amount per Serving:

- Calories 687
- % Daily Value*
- Total Fat 45.5g 58%
- Saturated Fat 6.4g 32%
- Cholesterol 0mg 0%
- Sodium 23mg 1%
- Total Carbohydrate 60.8g 22%
- Dietary Fiber 15.2g 54%
- Total Sugars 17.2g
- Protein 16.7g
- Vitamin D 0mcg 0%
- Calcium 118mg 9%
- Iron 6mg 33%
- Potassium 953mg 20%

Pegan Cauliflower Gnocchi in a Creamy Sauce

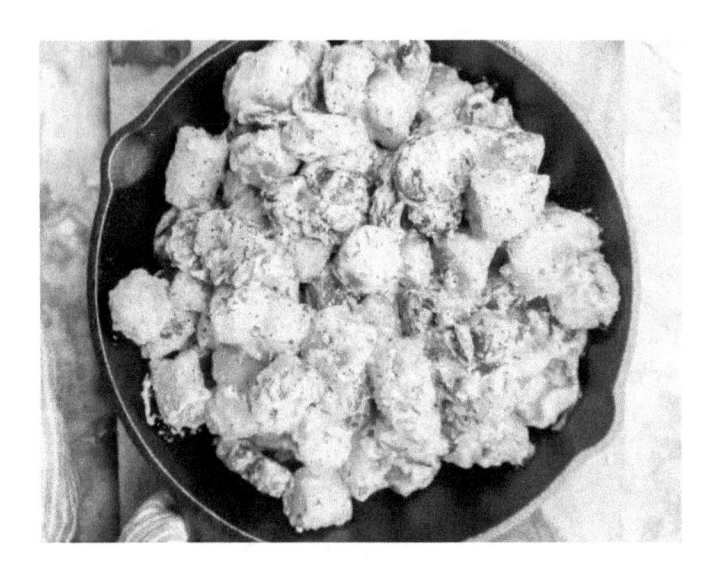

So good you'll forget it's good for you.

Makes: 4 servings.

Ingredients:

- 5 cups cauliflower, minced
- 1 cup cassava flour
- ½ teaspoon smoked paprika

Sauce

- 1 can coconut milk
- 5 cups spinach or kale
- 1 teaspoon garlic, minced
- ½ teaspoon lemon peel
- 1/3 teaspoon pepper

- 2 ½ tablespoons tapioca flour

Directions:

Steam cauliflower 5-7 minutes, ring out water, put in blender along with cassava flour and smoked paprika. Blend until mix is smooth.

Roll dough into 1-inch thick tube then cut into four segments, place three in the refrigerator.

Cut each segment into 1-inch pieces, drop them into boiling water and let rise to surface.

Once they have risen, transfer them to baking tray 20 minutes, turn over, cook another 30 minutes.

In skillet over medium-high heat whisk together coconut milk, spinach or kale, minced garlic, lemon peel, pepper, tapioca flour. Stirring continuously until smooth and thickens.

Remove from heat and add in spinach or kale and gnocchi.

Amount per Serving:

- *Calories 641*
- *% Daily Value**
- *Total Fat 29.3g 38%*
- *Saturated Fat 25.4g 127%*
- *Cholesterol 0mg 0%*
- *Sodium 196mg 9%*
- *Total Carbohydrate 92g 33%*

- *Dietary Fiber 10.4g 37%*
- *Total Sugars 7.2g*
- *Protein 6.8g*
- *Vitamin D 0mcg 0%*
- *Calcium 86mg 7%*
- *Iron 4mg 22%*
- *Potassium 916mg 19%*

Sweet Potato Gnocchi in an Herbed Dairy-Free Sauce

Throw some bell peppers or jalapenos in!

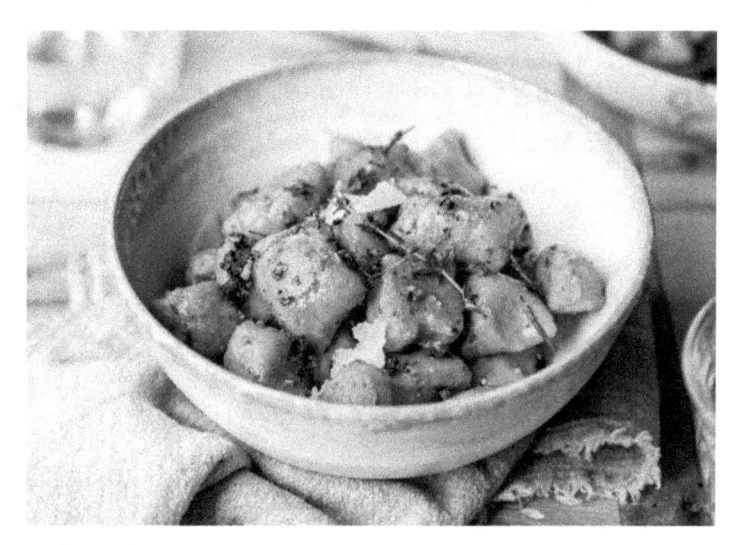

Makes: 2 servings.

Ingredients:

- 1 cup sweet potato mash
- ½ cup cassava or almond flour
- Olive oil
- 1 sprig parsley diced

Sauce

- 3 tablespoons unsalted butter or ghee
- 1 onion julienned
- 1 teaspoon garlic, minced
- ¾ can coconut milk

- 2 teaspoons tapioca flour
- 2 teaspoons rosemary, diced
- 2 teaspoons Italian oregano, diced
- 1/3 teaspoon red pepper flakes
- 1 cup spinach or kale

Directions:

Mix sweet potato mash and flour together until smooth. Roll into 1-inch thick tube and cut into 4 pieces. Stick three in the refrigerator.

Cut each segment into 1-inch pieces and stick on baking tray. Drizzle with olive oil and pieces of parsley.

Boil pieces until they rise to the top.

Transfer gnocchi pieces to skillet and cook over medium heat 1 minute or until each side is a golden brown.

In skillet let butter melt them add julienned onions. Turn heat to medium-low and let onions sweat 10 minutes.

Whisk in garlic and coconut milk, stirring constantly for 30 seconds. Whisk in tapioca flour, diced rosemary, diced oregano, red pepper flakes. Bring to a low boil for 1-2 minutes constantly stirring.

Remove from heat and stir in spinach/kale

Amount per Serving:

- *Calories 511*
- *% Daily Value**

- Total Fat 35g 45%
- Saturated Fat 23.9g 119%
- Cholesterol 15mg 5%
- Sodium 71mg 3%
- Total Carbohydrate 49.3g 18%
- Dietary Fiber 8g 29%
- Total Sugars 10.8g
- Protein 5.7g
- Vitamin D 0mcg 0%
- Calcium 87mg 7%
- Iron 7mg 37%
- Potassium 998mg 21%

Jalapeno Mango Salad

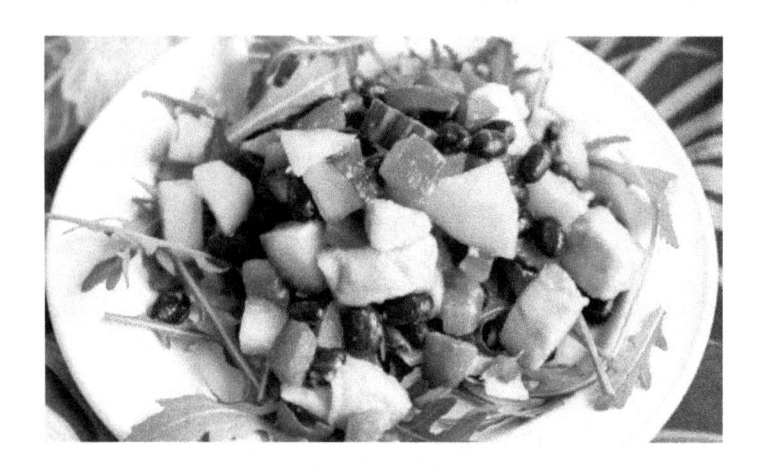

Try adding some rosemary!

Makes: 4 servings.

Ingredients:

- 1 medium Sweet Potato, chunked 2x2 pieces
- ¾ tablespoon Coconut Oil
- 1 cubed mango
- 1 cubed avocado
- 2/3 cup Cucumber, diced
- ½ tablespoon mint, thinly sliced
- ½ tablespoon cilantro, diced
- ½ tablespoon basil, diced

Sauce

- 2 tablespoons lime juice
- 2/3 cup extra virgin olive oil

- ¼ tsp pepper
- 1 cup red peppers, julienned
- 1 sliced jalapeno
- 1 banana pepper sliced

Directions:

Mix together lime juice, e.v.o.o, pepper, red peppers, jalapeno slices, banana pepper slices. Cover and chill.

Coat sweet potato chunks with coconut oil and cook 2-3 minutes per side to soften. Transfer to plate to cool then put in a bowl along with mango, avocado, cucumber slices, mint, cilantro, basil and stir.

Divide between four bowls and top each with vinaigrette.

Amount per Serving:

- *Calories 513*
- *% Daily Value**
- *Total Fat 46.6g 60%*
- *Saturated Fat 9.2g 46%*
- *Cholesterol 0mg 0%*
- *Sodium 78mg 3%*
- *Total Carbohydrate 28.3g 10%*
- *Dietary Fiber 6.6g 23%*
- *Total Sugars 16.2g*
- *Protein 3.2g*

- Vitamin D 0mcg 0%
- Calcium 29mg 2%
- Iron 2mg 11%
- Potassium 693mg 15

Toasted Coconut and Walnut Zoodle Salad with Baked Chicken Tenders

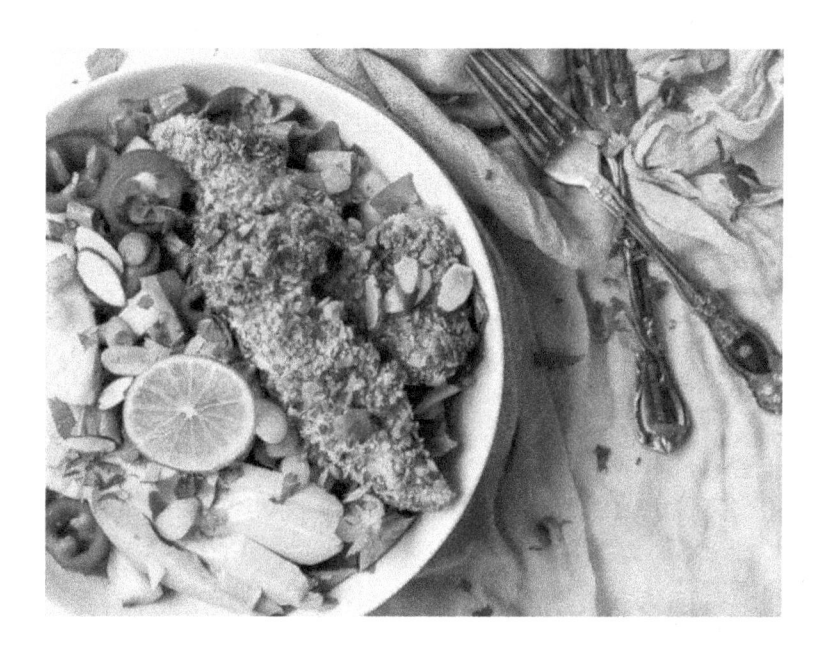

Make a great dipping sauce to accommodate these delicious tenders!

Makes: 2 serving.

Ingredients:

- 2/3 cup olive oil
- ½ teaspoon red or white wine
- 1/3 teaspoon lemon juice
- ½ teaspoon lemon peel
- 2 cups zucchini noodles
- 8 grape organic tomatoes

- ½ cup toasted coconut flakes
- ¼ cup toasted walnuts
- 8 lemon basil leaves, coarsely chopped OR 2 teaspoons organic Italian seasoning
- 6-8 organic chicken tenders
- 1 teaspoon Mexican seasoning like Tajin
- Olive oil for drizzling

Directions:

Preheat oven to 350 and prepare 9x11 dish.

Coat both sides of tenders with seasoning, lay on tray and drizzle with olive oil, bake 15 minutes, flip and repeat.

Mix together olive oil, wine, lemon juice, lemon peel; cover and chill.

In bowl combine zoodles, toasted coconut, toasted walnuts, chopped lemon basil leaves then top with vinaigrette and toss.

Divide amongst two plates and serve.

Amount per Serving:

- *Calories 945*
- *% Daily Value**
- *Total Fat 85.8g 110%*
- *Saturated Fat 16.8g 84%*
- *Cholesterol 31mg 10%*
- *Sodium 118mg 5%*
- *Total Carbohydrate 31.8g 12%*

- Dietary Fiber 7.7g 27%
- Total Sugars 18.5g
- Protein 19.6g
- Vitamin D 0mcg 0%
- Calcium 28mg 2%
- Iron 5mg 30%
- Potassium 1390mg 30

Pegan Quinoa Salad and Baked Tuna

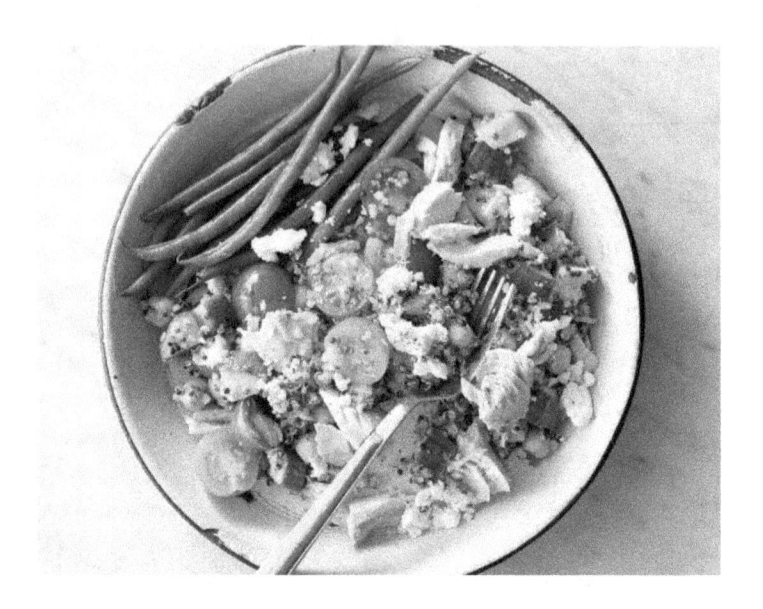

Also, great with fresh bay scallions.

Makes: 2 servings.

Ingredients:

- 2/3 cup quinoa, prepared ad directed
- ½ tablespoon red pepper infused olive oil
- ½ can organic whole kernel corn drained
- 3 pickled beets, quartered
- 1 teaspoon toasted coriander seeds
- 6 pickled jalapenos
- 1 ripe avocado peeled and sliced
- Juice of ½ lemon
- 2 filets tuna
- Salt and pepper

- ¼ cup coconut oil

Directions:

Preheat broiler to hi and prepare 9x11 dish.

In Dutch oven combine olive oil, corn, pickled beets, toasted coriander seeds, pickled jalapenos. Toss with prepared quinoa and warm through.

Sprinkle Tunas with salt and pepper then brush both sides with coconut oil. Place under broiler 4-5 minutes per-side.

Amount per Serving:

- Calories 787
- % Daily Value*
- Total Fat 51.3g 66%
- Saturated Fat 28.5g 142%
- Cholesterol 38mg 13%
- Sodium 284mg 12%
- Total Carbohydrate 55.2g 20%
- Dietary Fiber 11.9g 43%
- Total Sugars 9g
- Protein 30.5g
- Vitamin D 0mcg 0%
- Calcium 54mg 4%
- Iron 4mg 22%
- Potassium 1215mg 26%

Cauli-Bites

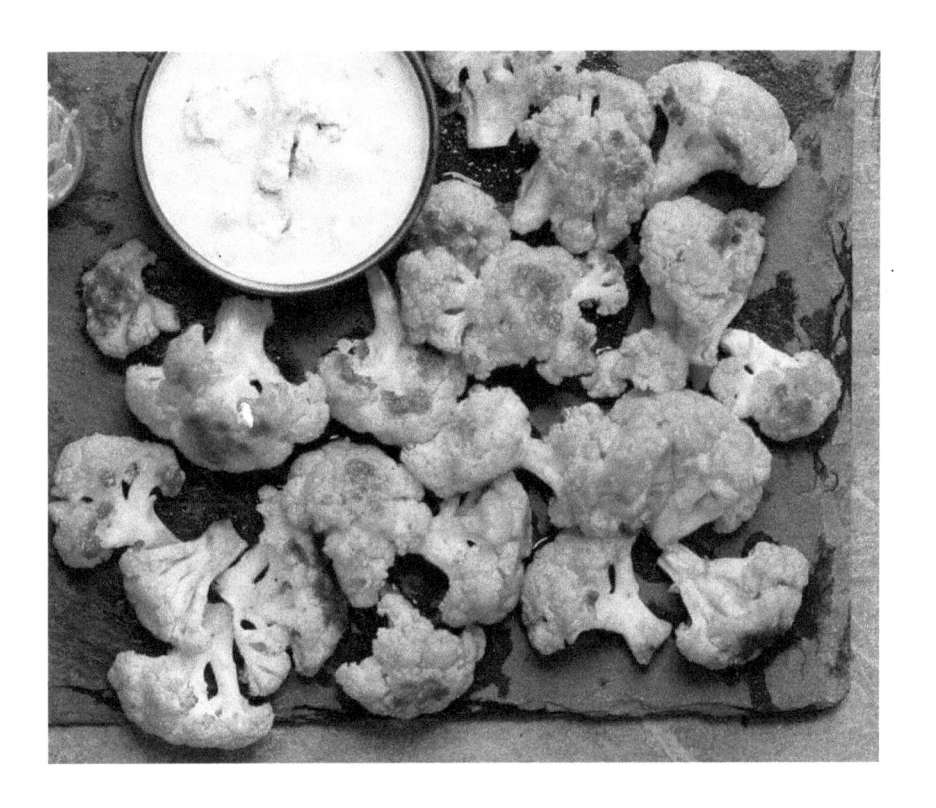

Great for making a treat out of last night leftovers.

Makes: 12 servings.

Ingredients:

- 4 cups cauliflower rice
- 2 tablespoon extra-virgin olive oil
- ½ teaspoon garlic, minced
- ½ teaspoon onion, minced
- 1 ½ teaspoon Italian seasoning

- 1 hamburger crumble or 1 ½ cup ground beef, browned and drained (optional)

Directions:

Preheat oven to 350 and prepare muffin tin.

Mix together cauliflower rice, e.v.o.o, minced garlic, diced onion, Italian seasoning, ground beef or crumble.

Press into muffin tins and bake 30 minutes.

Store in airtight container in refrigerator and will keep 3-5 days.

Amount per Serving:

- *Calories 53*
- *% Daily Value**
- *Total Fat 3.6g 5%*
- *Saturated Fat 0.8g 4%*
- *Cholesterol 6mg 2%*
- *Sodium 45mg 2%*
- *Total Carbohydrate 2.3g 1%*
- *Dietary Fiber 0g 0%*
- *Total Sugars 1.4g*
- *Protein 3.2g*
- *Vitamin D 0mcg 0%*
- *Calcium 1mg 0%*
- *Iron 0mg 1%*

- *Potassium 26mg 1%*

Crispy Baked Chicken with Sweet Potato & Broccoli Tots

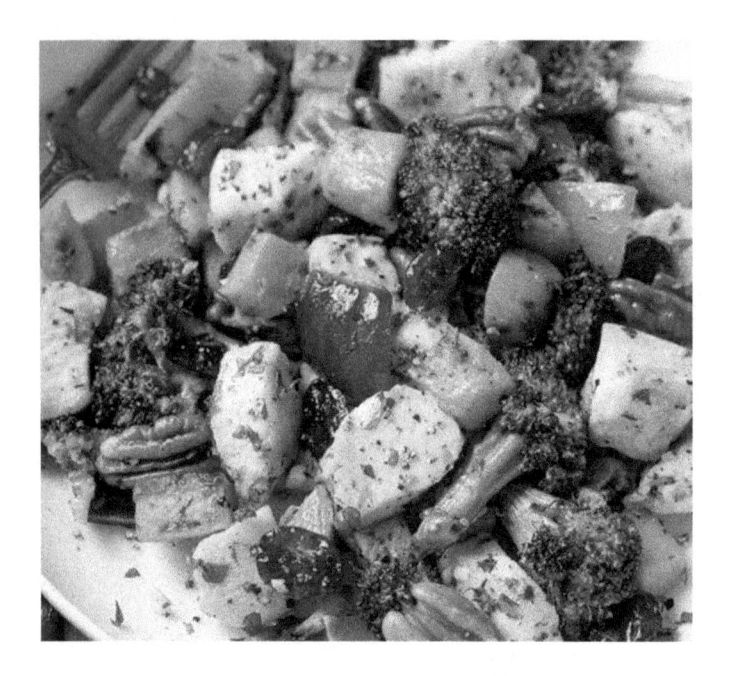

Also, great with a meatless burger!

Makes: 2 servings.

Ingredients:

- 2 3 oz. chicken patties
- 1 cup organic breadcrumbs or crushed cornflakes
- 2 cups sweet potato mash
- 2 cups broccoli mash
- 1 tablespoon paprika
- ½ tablespoon garlic powder and parsley

Directions:

Preheat oven to 425 and prepare medium sized baking dish.

Coat chicken patties with breadcrumbs, spray with olive oil, bake 35-40 minutes.

Blend together sweet potato, broccoli, paprika, garlic powder and parsley.

Using hands form into tater tots and fry in coconut oil 2-3 minutes per side.

Amount per Serving:

- Calories 727
- % Daily Value*
- Total Fat 24g 31%
- Saturated Fat 4.7g 24%
- Cholesterol 45mg 15%
- Sodium 1016mg 44%
- Total Carbohydrate 102.1g 37%
- Dietary Fiber 14g 50%
- Total Sugars 18.2g
- Protein 28.6g
- Vitamin D 0mcg 0%
- Calcium 175mg 13%
- Iron 12mg 67%
- Potassium 1673mg 36%

Mexican Sweet Tater Tots with Coconut-Cinnamon Pork Chops

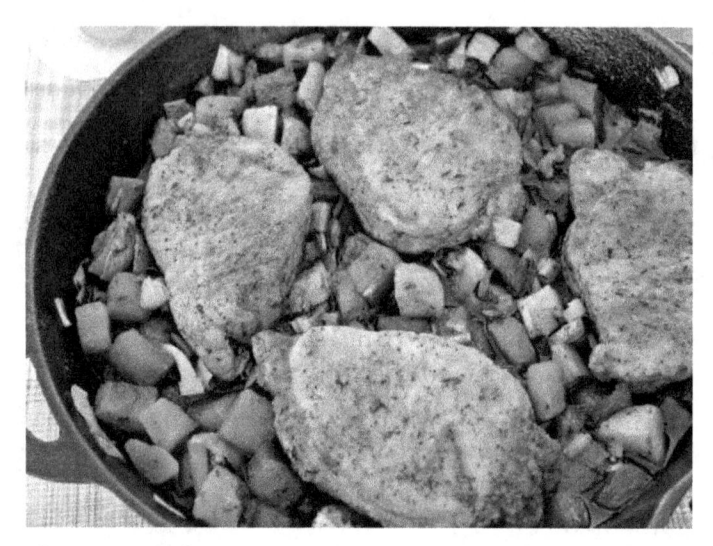

Try substituting the sweet potato mash with cauliflower mash!

Makes: 2 servings.

Ingredients:

- 1 tablespoon coconut oil
- 2 thin pork chops
- Cinnamon for sprinkling
- 4 cup sweet potato mash
- 1 tablespoon chili powder
- 1 tablespoon paprika
- 1 tablespoon cayenne pepper
- ½ tablespoon cumin
- ½ tablespoon garlic powder and parsley
- Coconut oil for frying OR olive oil infused with red pepper

Directions:

In skillet cook pork chops in coconut oil transfer to paper towel lined plates.

Mix together sweet potato, chili powder, paprika, cayenne powder, cumin, garlic powder & parsley.

With hands form into tater tots and fry in oil 2-3 minutes per side.

Before plating dust both sides of pork chops with cinnamon.

Amount per Serving:

- *Calories 230*
- *% Daily Value**
- *Total Fat 11.7g 15%*
- *Saturated Fat 7.2g 36%*
- *Cholesterol 60mg 20%*
- *Sodium 275mg 12%*
- *Total Carbohydrate 8.8g 3%*
- *Dietary Fiber 3.6g 13%*
- *Total Sugars 2.7g*
- *Protein 23.6g*
- *Vitamin D 0mcg 0%*
- *Calcium 37mg 3%*
- *Iron 3mg 14%*
- *Potassium 243mg 5%*

Easy Grilled Veggie Turkey Sliders

Try it with ground pork or as a veggie burger!

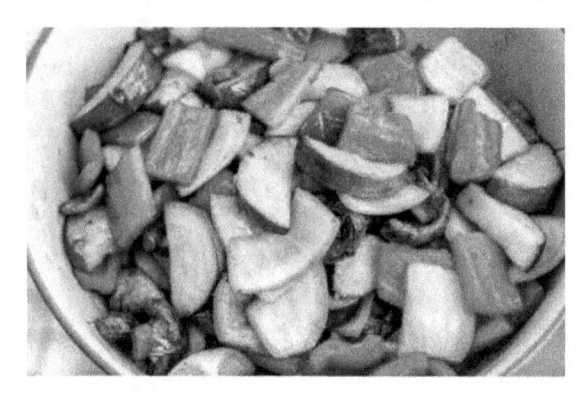

Makes: 5-7 servings.

Ingredients:

- ½ lbs. ground turkey
- 1/3 cup shredded carrots
- 1/3 cup shredded beets
- 1/3 cup zucchini
- ½ teaspoon garlic, minced
- 1 teaspoon onion, minced
- 1 teaspoon ginger, minced
- ½ teaspoon brown sugar
- ½ teaspoon black pepper
- ½ teaspoon paprika

Directions:

Mix together ground turkey, shredded carrots, shredded beets, shredded zucchini, minced garlic, minced onion, minced ginger, brown sugar, black pepper, paprika.

Using hands form into 3 oz. patties, grill over medium-high heat 4-5 minutes per side.

Amount per Serving:

- *Calories 85*
- *% Daily Value**
- *Total Fat 4.2g 5%*
- *Saturated Fat 0.7g 4%*
- *Cholesterol 39mg 13%*
- *Sodium 53mg 2%*
- *Total Carbohydrate 2.6g 1%*
- *Dietary Fiber 0.6g 2%*
- *Total Sugars 1.5g*
- *Protein 10.7g*
- *Vitamin D 0mcg 0%*
- *Calcium 16mg 1%*
- *Iron 1mg 5%*
- *Potassium 179mg 4%*

Creamy Dairy-Free Veggie Soup

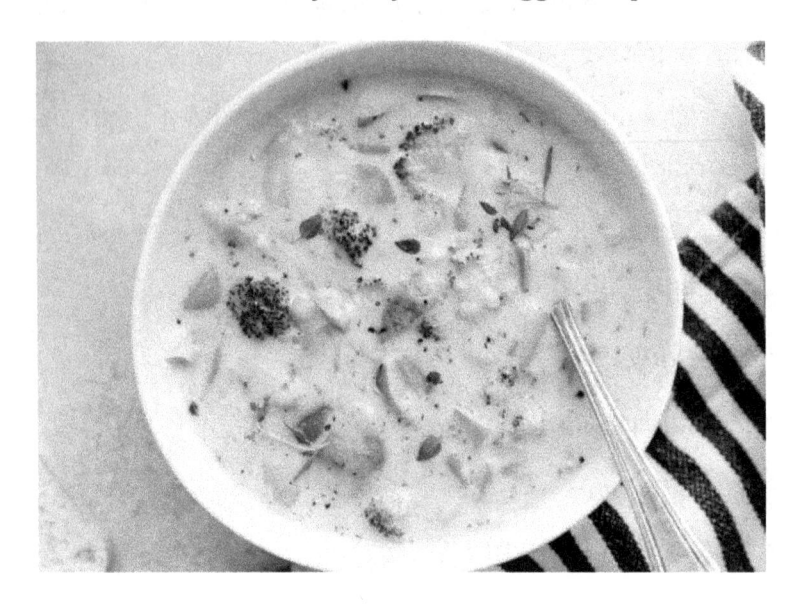

Minced turmeric is a great addition!

Makes: 4 servings.

Ingredients:

- 1 head of cauliflower, chopped
- 1/3 cup walnuts
- ½ cup carrots chopped
- 1/3 cup cremini mushrooms, sliced
- ¼ cup onion, minced
- 1 tsp garlic, minced
- 4 tablespoons olive oil infused with basil
- 2 tablespoon cracked black pepper
- ½ tablespoon parsley, diced

Directions:

In Dutch oven add infused oil and sauté carrots, cremini mushrooms, minced onions, minced garlic.

In blender chop cauliflower and walnuts, then add to Dutch oven. Stir in pepper and parsley. Simmer 7-10 minutes.

Amount per Serving:

- Calories 220
- % Daily Value*
- Total Fat 20.3g 26%
- Saturated Fat 2.4g 12%
- Cholesterol 0mg 0%
- Sodium 32mg 1%
- Total Carbohydrate 9.1g 3%
- Dietary Fiber 3.8g 14%
- Total Sugars 2.8g
- Protein 4.6g
- Vitamin D 0mcg 0%
- Calcium 44mg 3%
- Iron 2mg 9%
- Potassium 382mg 8%

Roasted Veggies with Easy Homemade Tahini Sauce

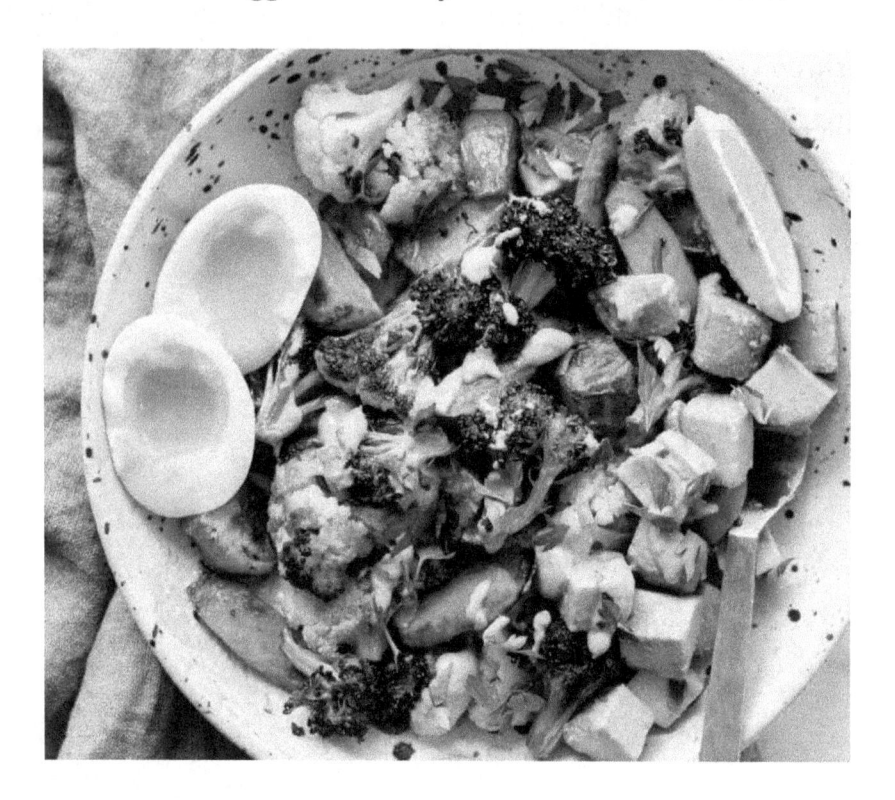

Also great with a curry sauce!

Makes: 2 servings.

Ingredients:

- 2 cups broccoli trees
- 2 cups baby carrots
- 1 cup plum tomatoes, halved
- 2 cups string beans
- Olive oil spray
- 1 bunch parsley, approx. 1 cup

- 2 teaspoons lemon juice
- 2 teaspoons extra virgin olive oil
- 1 teaspoon garlic, minced
- 2 tablespoons tahini

Directions:

Preheat oven to 400 and line baking sheet with parchment paper.

Layout broccoli trees, baby carrots, halved plum tomatoes and mist with olive oil. Bake 20 minutes.

Blend parsley, lemon juice, extra virgin olive oil, minced garlic, tahini together.

Pour sauce over roasted veggie's and enjoy

Amount per Serving:

- *Calories 220*
- *% Daily Value**
- *Total Fat 13.4g 17%*
- *Saturated Fat 1.9g 10%*
- *Cholesterol 0mg 0%*
- *Sodium 70mg 3%*
- *Total Carbohydrate 22.6g 8%*
- *Dietary Fiber 8.7g 31%*
- *Total Sugars 6.9g*
- *Protein 8.5g*
- *Vitamin D 0mcg 0%*

- *Calcium 169mg 13%*
- *Iron 4mg 22%*
- *Potassium 804mg 17%*

Zoodle Noodle Salad with Easy Basil Dressing

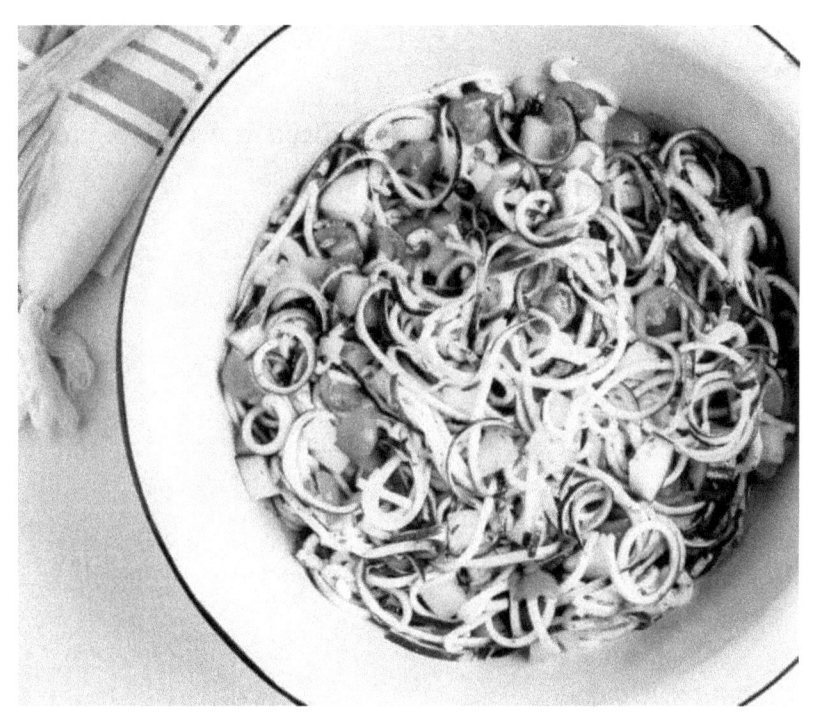

Also, great with sweet potato noodles!

Makes: 4 servings.

Ingredients:

- 2 cups zoodles
- 1 cup scallions, chopped
- 1 red bell pepper, diced
- 1 cup sliced mushrooms
- 2 tablespoons diced Italian oregano
- 1 ½ tablespoon extra-virgin olive oil
- ½ tablespoon balsamic vinegar

- 2 tablespoons lemon juice
- 1 tablespoon basil, chopped
- 1 teaspoon minced garlic

Directions:

Mix together zoodles, chopped scallions, diced red bell pepper, sliced mushrooms, diced Italian oregano,

Mix together e.v.o.o, balsamic vinegar, basil, garlic.

Amount per Serving:

- *Calories 84*
- *% Daily Value**
- *Total Fat 5.8g 7%*
- *Saturated Fat 0.9g 5%*
- *Cholesterol 0mg 0%*
- *Sodium 13mg 1%*
- *Total Carbohydrate 8.2g 3%*
- *Dietary Fiber 2.8g 10%*
- *Total Sugars 3.5g*
- *Protein 2.3g*
- *Vitamin D 63mcg 315%*
- *Calcium 66mg 5%*
- *Iron 2mg 12%*
- *Potassium 362mg 8%*
- *Desserts & Snacks*

Pegan Friendly Apple Crisps

Great for special occasions!

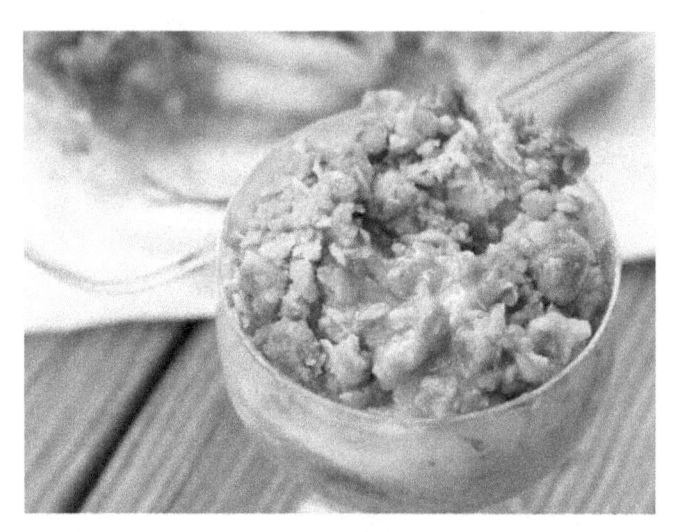

Makes: 4 servings.

Ingredients:

- 1 large can apple pie filling
- 1 teaspoon apple pie seasoning
- 3 – 3 ½ cups of gluten free rice or corn squares (such as Chex)
- Whipped topping

Directions:

Mix seasoning & filling together and split between four bowls; topping each with cereal and whipped topping.

Amount per Serving:

- Calories 317
- % Daily Value*
- Total Fat 7.2g 9%
- Saturated Fat 4.2g 21%
- Cholesterol 23mg 8%
- Sodium 326mg 14%
- Total Carbohydrate 62.3g 23%
- Dietary Fiber 2.2g 8%
- Total Sugars 25.2g
- Protein 2.6g
- Vitamin D 0mcg 2%
- Calcium 111mg 9%
- Iron 7mg 40%
- Potassium 137mg 3%

G.F. Chocolate and Peanut Butter No-Bake Granola Bites

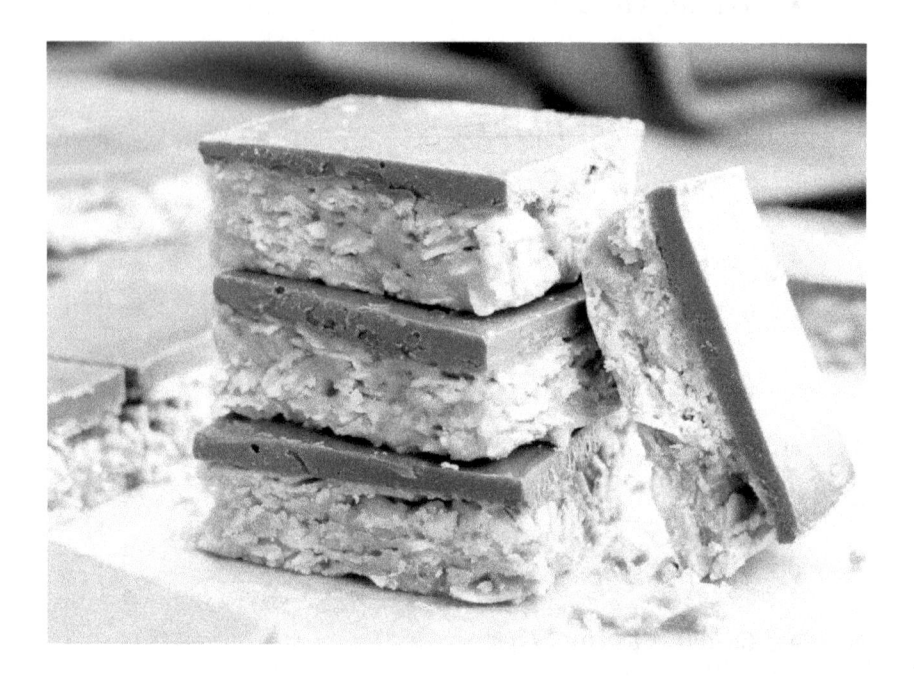

Easy on the go treats!

Makes: approx. 10 - 13 servings.

Ingredients:

- 2 tablespoon brown sugar
- 2 tablespoon organic honey
- 1/3 cup g.f peanut butter
- ½ cup roasted unsalted peanuts
- 1 bag flavored g.f. cereal such as Chex Granola Mixed Berry Almond
- ¼ cup chocolate chips

Directions:

Preheat oven to and line baking tray with parchment.

In a bowl mix together cereal, chocolate chips, and peanuts.

Add to saucepan brown sugar, honey, peanut butter and boil one minute.

Add melted peanut butter mixture to cereal mix and stir.

With spoon or ice cream scoop, lay out granola bites 2-inches apart then chill in refrigerator 30 minutes.

Amount per Serving:

- Calories 131
- % Daily Value*
- Total Fat 8.3g 11%
- Saturated Fat 2.1g 10%
- Cholesterol 1mg 0%
- Sodium 63mg 3%
- Total Carbohydrate 11.7g 4%
- Dietary Fiber 1.2g 4%
- Total Sugars 7.9g
- Protein 4.2g
- Vitamin D 0mcg 0%
- Calcium 24mg 2%
- Iron 2mg 11%
- Potassium 119mg 3%

Vanilla Bean and Strawberry Dessert

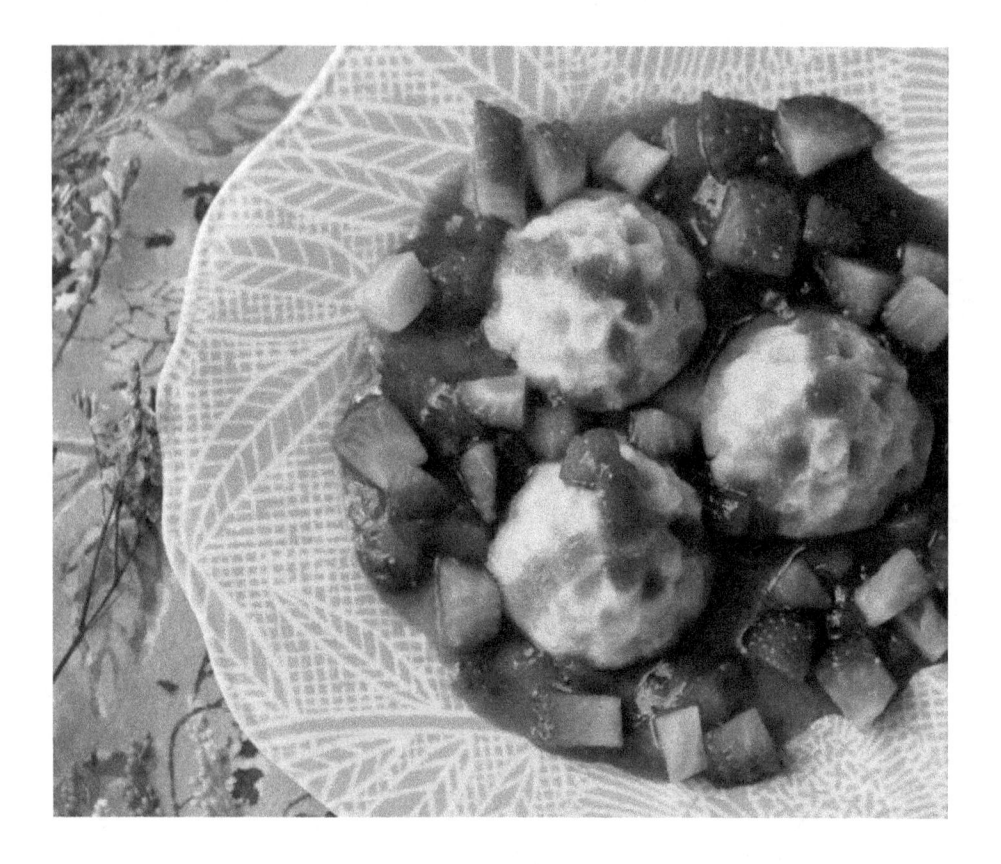

This syrup is also good for pancakes and on bananas!

Makes: approx. 2 servings.

Ingredients:

- 2 cups chopped strawberries, divided
- Maple syrup, for drizzling
- ½ cup toasted coconut, flaked
- 1 vanilla bean, seeds removed
- ½ cup crushed walnuts

- 4 cups whipped topping, divided
- 2 mint or basil leaves, torn (optional)

Directions:

Preheat oven to 400 and line baking tray with parchment paper.

Layout strawberries on tray, drizzle with maple syrup, bake 18-22 minutes.

Meanwhile toasted coconut and walnuts in skillet set over med.-low heat.

Put glazed strawberries, toasted coconut and waffles on top of whipped topping and torn herb leaves.

Amount per Serving:

- *Calories 715*
- *% Daily Value**
- *Total Fat 58.9g 76%*
- *Saturated Fat 29.5g 147%*
- *Cholesterol 91mg 30%*
- *Sodium 167mg 7%*
- *Total Carbohydrate 42g 15%*
- *Dietary Fiber 8.6g 31%*
- *Total Sugars 25.4g*
- *Protein 13.7g*
- *Vitamin D 0mcg 0%*
- *Calcium 172mg 13%*

- *Iron 7mg 41%*
- *Potassium 724mg 15%*

Pegan Nutella

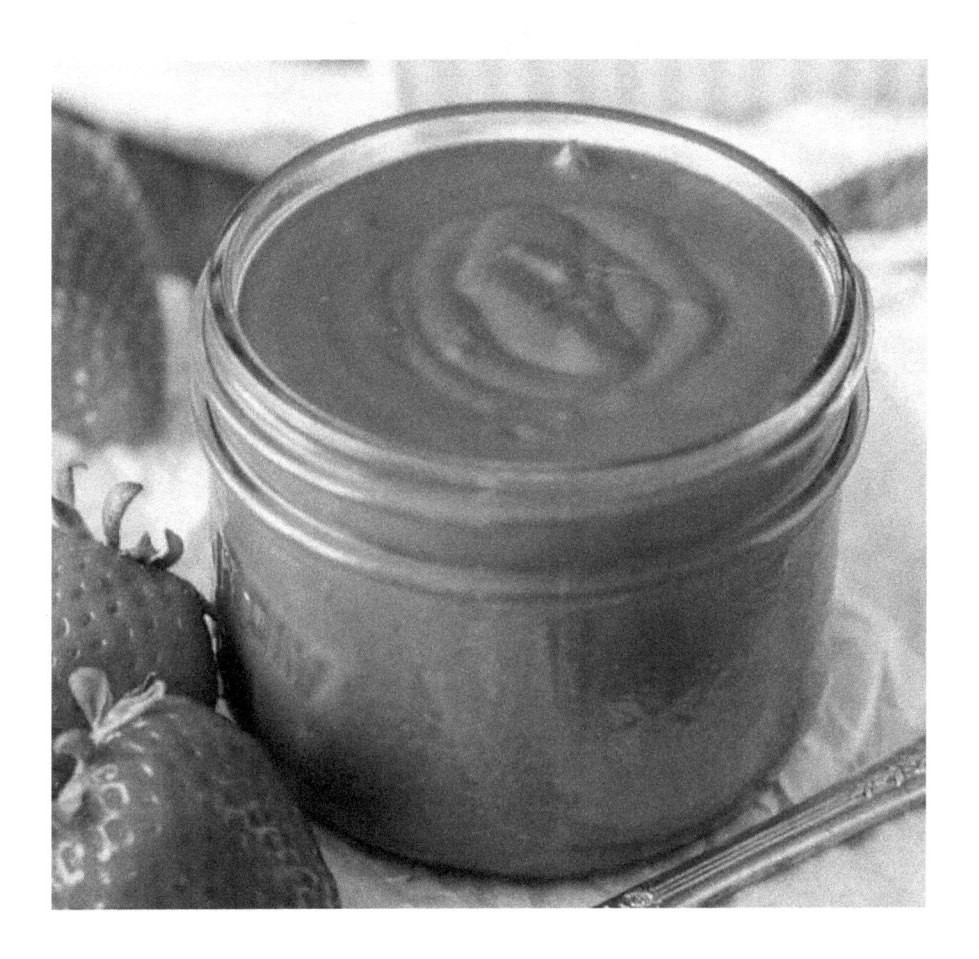

Great for homemade granolas!

Makes: approx. 1 – 1 ½ cups.

Ingredients:

- ½ tablespoon coconut oil
- 1 ½ tablespoon sunflower seed butter

- 2 tablespoon unsweetened cacao powder or blend carob pieces till a powder
- 2 T organic honey, agave, or sugar-free maple syrup

Directions:

Mix together coconut oil; sunflower butter; cacao powder or carob powder; honey, agave, or syrup.

If too thick add small amount of sunflower butter or coconut oil.

Amount per Serving:

- *Calories 263*
- *% Daily Value**
- *Total Fat 17.1g 22%*
- *Saturated Fat 8.5g 43%*
- *Cholesterol 0mg 0%*
- *Sodium 6mg 0%*
- *Total Carbohydrate 24.6g 9%*
- *Dietary Fiber 2g 7%*
- *Total Sugars 17.3g*
- *Protein 4.4g*
- *Vitamin D 0mcg 0%*
- *Calcium 36mg 3%*
- *Iron 2mg 10%*
- *Potassium 20mg 0%*

Pegan Friendly Cheesecake Bites in Caramel Sauce

Grocery stores are selling more and more organics, so finding these ingredients shouldn't be a problem!

Makes: 12.

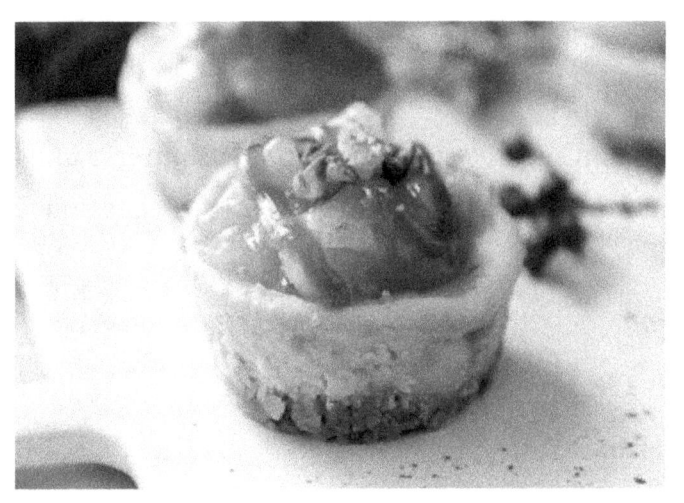

Ingredients:

- ¾ cup pitted dates
- ¾ raw almonds
- 1 cup + 1 tablespoon raw cashews (soaked overnight, then drained)
- 1 can coconut milk
- 3 tablespoons maple syrup
- 2 tablespoons melted coconut oil
- ¾ cup coconut palm sugar
- ½ coconut milk
- 1/3 cup honey

- 4 tablespoon grass-fed butter or ghee
- ½ teaspoon vanilla extract

Directions:

Prepare muffin-tin.

For crust- blend together pitted dates and almonds. Using a spoon, place a heaping amount in each muffin tin then press firmly down.

For filling- Blend together cashews, coconut cream, syrup, & 2 teaspoon coconut oil. Pour into tins and freeze 5 hours.

For caramel sauce- palm sugar, coconut milk, honey, butter, vanilla extract. Warm in pot over medium heat. Drizzle over cheesecake bites and enjoy!

Amount per Serving:

- *Calories 1929*
- *% Daily Value**
- *Total Fat 119.4g 153%*
- *Saturated Fat 77.1g 385%*
- *Cholesterol 22mg 7%*
- *Sodium 309mg 13%*
- *Total Carbohydrate 226.4g 82%*
- *Dietary Fiber 12.9g 46%*
- *Total Sugars 172.2g*
- *Protein 19.2g*
- *Vitamin D 0mcg 0%*

- *Calcium 133mg 10%*
- *Iron 11mg 63%*
- *Potassium 1686mg 36%*

Cool Mint Coconut Chia Pudding

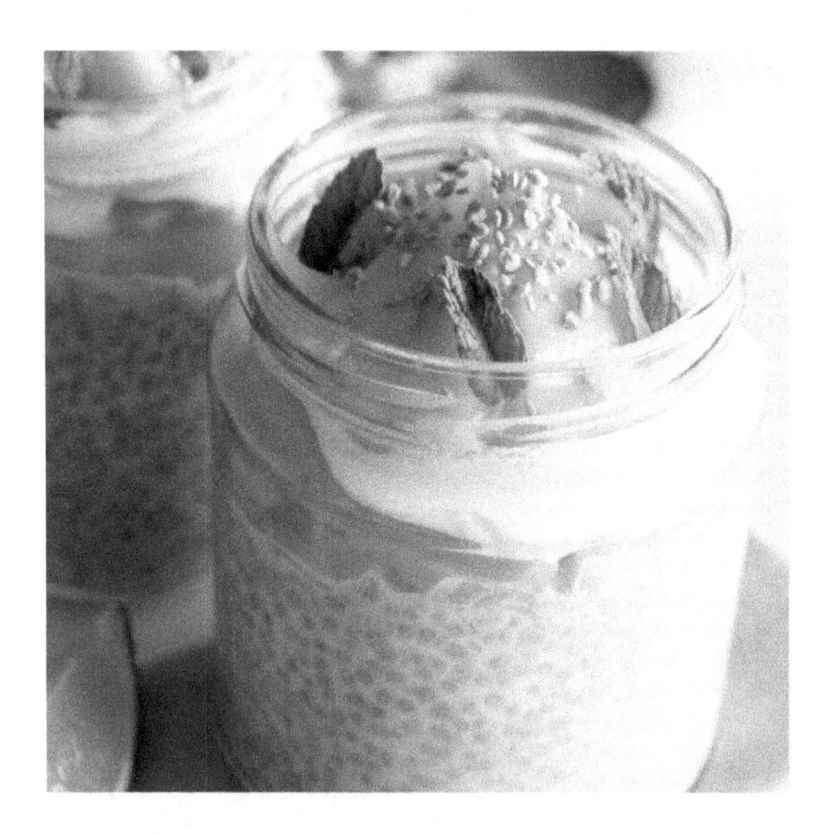

Mint and coconut is a great combo!

Makes: 2 servings.

Ingredients:

- 1 cup almond milk
- ¾ cup coconut milk
- 1 Tbsp maple syrup
- ½ tsp lime juice
- ½ tablespoon mint flavored extract

- ⅓ cup chia seeds
- ¼ cup coconut flakes
- 1 ½ cup mango

Directions:

Mix together almond milk, coconut milk, syrup, lime juice, mint extract, chia seeds. Let rest at room temp 10 minutes then cover and sit in refrigerator 4-8 hours.

Toast coconut in skillet over medium-high heat 2 minutes.

Stir toasted coconut and mango on top of pudding and enjoy.

Amount per Serving:

- *Calories 637*
- *% Daily Value**
- *Total Fat 56.6g 73%*
- *Saturated Fat 49.8g 249%*
- *Cholesterol 0mg 0%*
- *Sodium 37mg 2%*
- *Total Carbohydrate 37.5g 14%*
- *Dietary Fiber 5.6g 20%*
- *Total Sugars 27.7g*
- *Protein 6.4g*
- *Vitamin D 0mcg 0%*
- *Calcium 62mg 5%*
- *Iron 7mg 41%*

- *Potassium 841mg 18%*

Pegan Marshmallow Mint Brownies

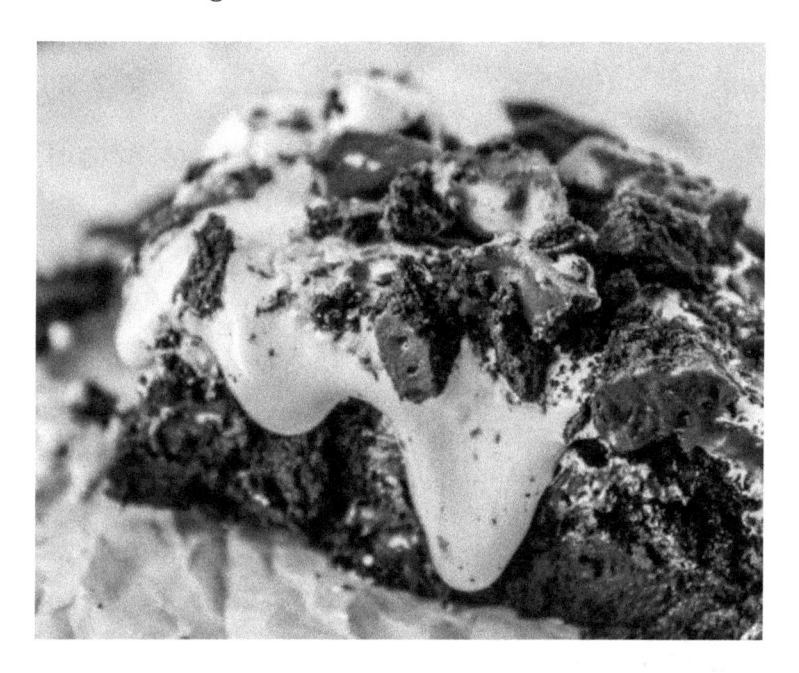

For extra mint try minty Choco chips!

Makes: 9 servings.

Ingredients:

- 1/3 cup coconut oil, melted
- 4 heaping tablespoons cocoa powder
- 2 oz unsweetened bakers' chocolate
- 2/3 cup honey or agave
- 2 large eggs, room temperature
- 1 teaspoon vanilla
- ¼ cup coconut flour
- 2/3 teaspoon mint flavored extract

- 3 cups large marshmallows OR 1 cup mini marshmallows melted

Directions:

Preheat oven to 350 and prepare a 9x9 dish by lining it with parchment paper.

In saucepan over medium heat melt coconut oil, cocoa powder, and unsweetened Bakers' chocolate. Stirring until there are no lumps.

Add in beating well after each addition: honey, eggs, vanilla, coconut flour, mint extract, melted marshmallows.

Pour into 9x9 pan and bake 20-25 minutes; store in airtight container in refrigerator.

Amount per Serving:

- *Calories 1088*
- *% Daily Value**
- *Total Fat 58.6g 75%*
- *Saturated Fat 43.8g 219%*
- *Cholesterol 164mg 55%*
- *Sodium 109mg 5%*
- *Total Carbohydrate 151.6g 55%*
- *Dietary Fiber 14.2g 51%*
- *Total Sugars 113.7g*
- *Protein 13.8g*

- *Vitamin D 15mcg 77%*
- *Calcium 72mg 6%*
- *Iron 8mg 44%*
- *Potassium 629mg 13%*

Pegan Peanut Butter Brownies

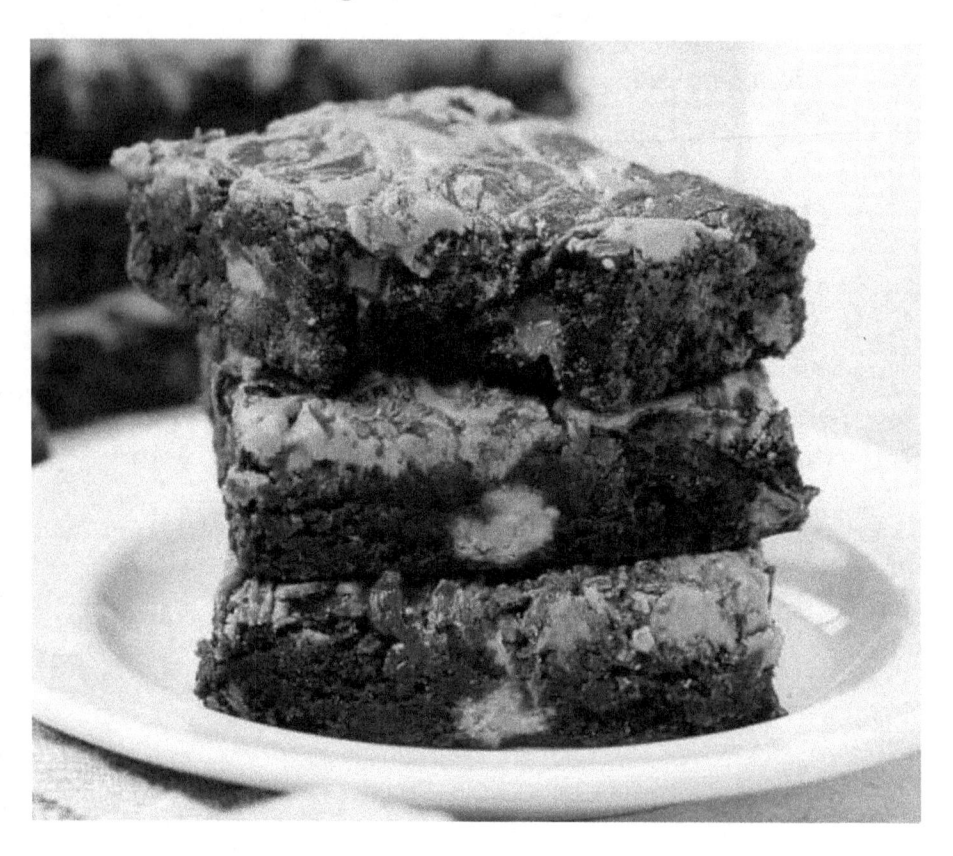

Dairy free deliciousness!

Makes: 9 servings.

Ingredients:

- 1/3 cup coconut oil, melted
- 4 heaping tablespoons cocoa powder
- 2 oz unsweetened bakers' chocolate
- 2/3 cup honey or agave
- 2 large eggs, room temperature

- 1 teaspoon vanilla
- ¼ cup coconut flour
- 1 cup natural or organic peanut butter, melted
- 1 package peanut butter chips

Directions:

Preheat oven to 350 and prepare a 9x9 dish by lining it with parchment paper.

In saucepan over medium heat melt coconut oil, cocoa powder, and unsweetened Bakers' chocolate. Stirring until there are no lumps.

Add in beating well after each addition: honey, eggs, vanilla, coconut flour, melted peanut butter.

Mix in peanut butter chips.

Pour into 9x9 pan and bake 20-25 minutes; store in airtight container in refrigerator.

Amount per Serving:

- *Calories 1088*
- *% Daily Value**
- *Total Fat 58.6g 75%*
- *Saturated Fat 43.8g 219%*
- *Cholesterol 164mg 55%*
- *Sodium 109mg 5%*
- *Total Carbohydrate 151.6g 55%*
- *Dietary Fiber 14.2g 51%*

- *Total Sugars 113.7g*
- *Protein 13.8g*
- *Vitamin D 15mcg 77%*
- *Calcium 72mg 6%*
- *Iron 8mg 44%*
- *Potassium 629mg 13%*

Pegan Peanut Butter & Marshmallow Mint Brownies

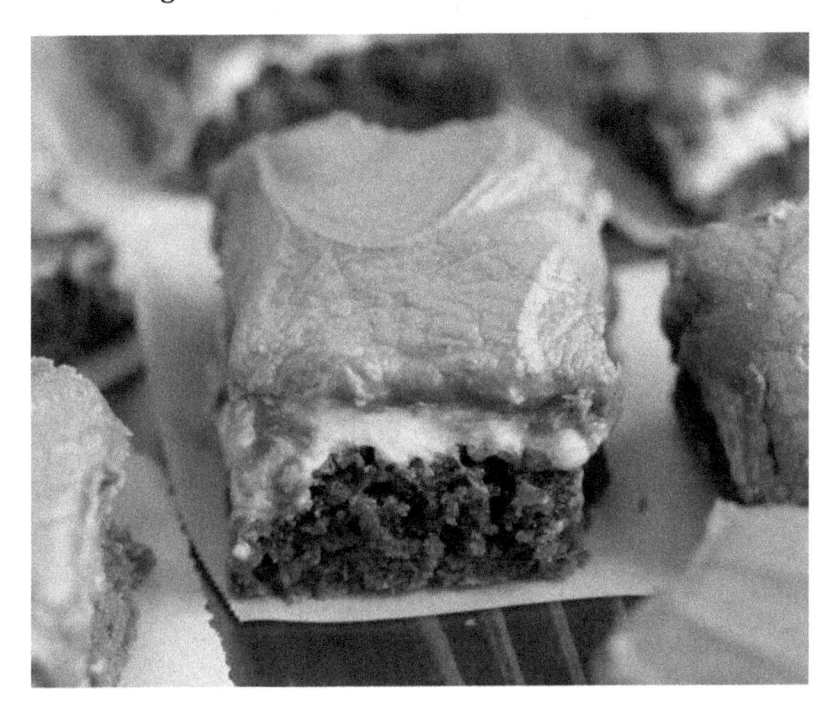

Great treat for kids!

Makes: 9 servings.

Ingredients:

- 1/3 cup coconut oil, melted
- 4 heaping tablespoons cocoa powder
- 2 oz unsweetened bakers' chocolate
- 2/3 cup honey or agave
- 2 large eggs, room temperature
- 1 teaspoon vanilla
- ¼ cup coconut flour
- 1 teaspoon mint flavored extract

- 1 package mini marshmallows
- 1 12 oz. package organic peanut butter chips

Directions:

Preheat oven to 350 and prepare a 9x9 dish by lining it with parchment paper.

In saucepan over medium heat melt coconut oil, cocoa powder, and unsweetened Bakers' chocolate. Stirring until there are no lumps.

Add in beating well after each addition: honey, eggs, vanilla, coconut flour, mint extract, mini marshmallows, peanut butter chips.

Pour into 9x9 pan and bake 23-28 minutes; store in airtight container in refrigerator.

Amount per Serving:

- *Calories 1088*
- *% Daily Value**
- *Total Fat 58.6g 75%*
- *Saturated Fat 43.8g 219%*
- *Cholesterol 164mg 55%*
- *Sodium 109mg 5%*
- *Total Carbohydrate 151.6g 55%*
- *Dietary Fiber 14.2g 51%*
- *Total Sugars 113.7g*

- *Protein 13.8g*
- *Vitamin D 15mcg 77%*
- *Calcium 72mg 6%*
- *Iron 8mg 44%*
- *Potassium 629mg 13%*

Pagan Friendly Chocolate Loaf

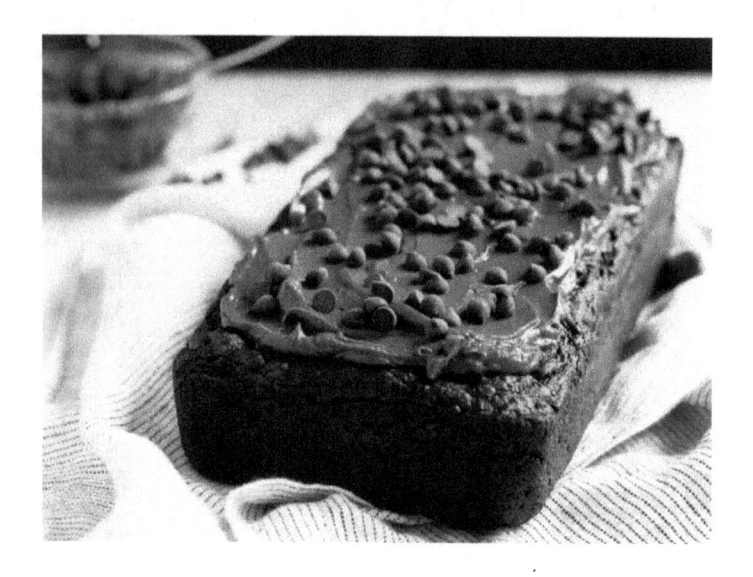

Great for a Valentine's Day treat.

Makes: approx. 10 slices.

Ingredients:

- 1 ¼ cup beets
- 1 1/3 cups blanched almond flour
- 1/3 cup + 1 tablespoon coconut flour
- ¼ cup + 2 teaspoons cocoa powder
- ½ teaspoon baking soda
- 2/3 cup coconut milk
- 3 eggs
- 1 egg yolk
- ½ cup maple syrup
- 1 teaspoon vanilla extract

- 1 package semi-sweet chocolate chips

Directions:

Preheat oven to 350 and line loaf pan with parchment paper.

Microwave beets 4-5 minutes then set aside.

Whisk together almond & coconut flour, cocoa powder, baking powder.

Blend until smooth: coconut milk, eggs, yolk, syrup, vanilla extract, beets.

Pour liquid ingredients into dry and stir. Pour into loaf pan and bake 45-55 minutes.

Seal leftovers in airtight container in refrigerator will keep 1 week.

Amount per Serving:

- *Calories 218*
- *% Daily Value**
- *Total Fat 13.4g 17%*
- *Saturated Fat 5g 25%*
- *Cholesterol 70mg 23%*
- *Sodium 98mg 4%*
- *Total Carbohydrate 19.6g 7%*
- *Dietary Fiber 4.4g 16%*
- *Total Sugars 10.8g*
- *Protein 6.6g*
- *Vitamin D 6mcg 32%*

- *Calcium 26mg 2%*
- *Iron 1mg 6%*
- *Potassium 174mg*

Raspberry Frosting

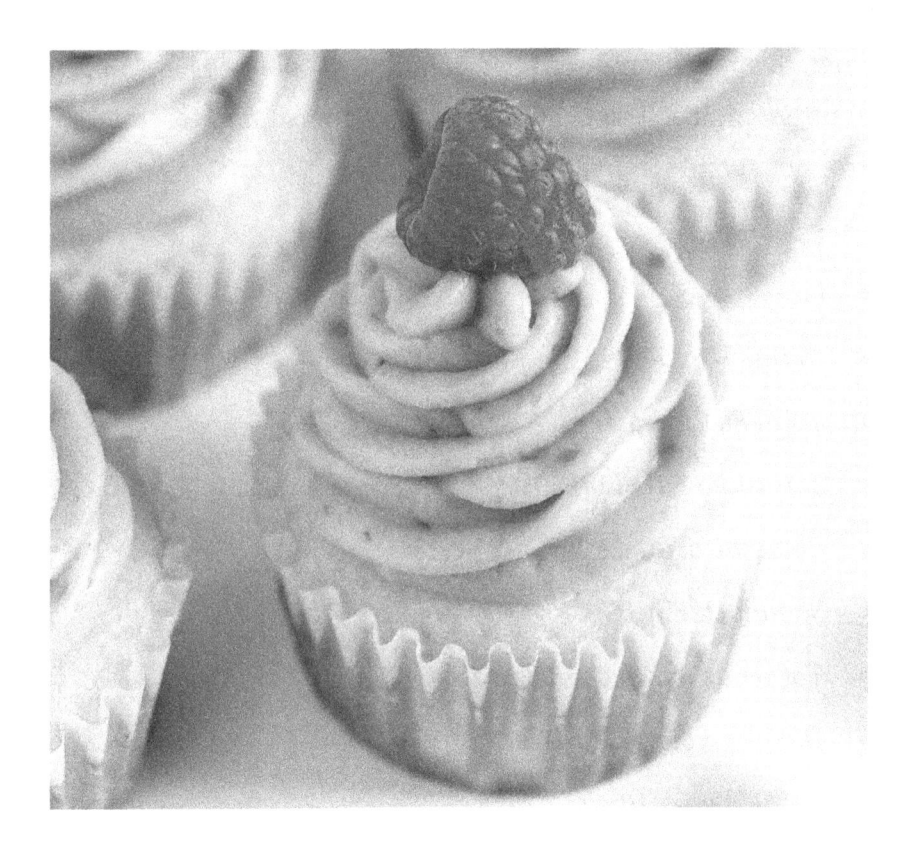

for various pastries!

Makes: approx. 1 cup

Ingredients:

- 2/3 cup chilled or frozen raspberries
- ¾ tablespoon +1 teaspoon maple syrup
- ½ cup coconut butter
- ½ tablespoon mint extract
- 2-3 mint leaves for top

- 2 tablespoons cornstarch

Directions:

In small pot over medium-low heat combine raspberries, syrup, coconut butter, mint extract. Stir constantly for 2 minutes then remove from heat and stir in cornstarch.

Amount per Serving:

- Calories 467
- % Daily Value*
- Total Fat 36.3g 47%
- Saturated Fat 32g 160%
- Cholesterol 0mg 0%
- Sodium 22mg 1%
- Total Carbohydrate 31.2g 11%
- Dietary Fiber 12.7g 46%
- Total Sugars 10.3g
- Protein 4.5g
- Vitamin D 0mcg 0%
- Calcium 15mg 1%
- Iron 0mg 2%
- Potassium 77mg 2%

Breakfast

Apple Pie Pegan Pancakes

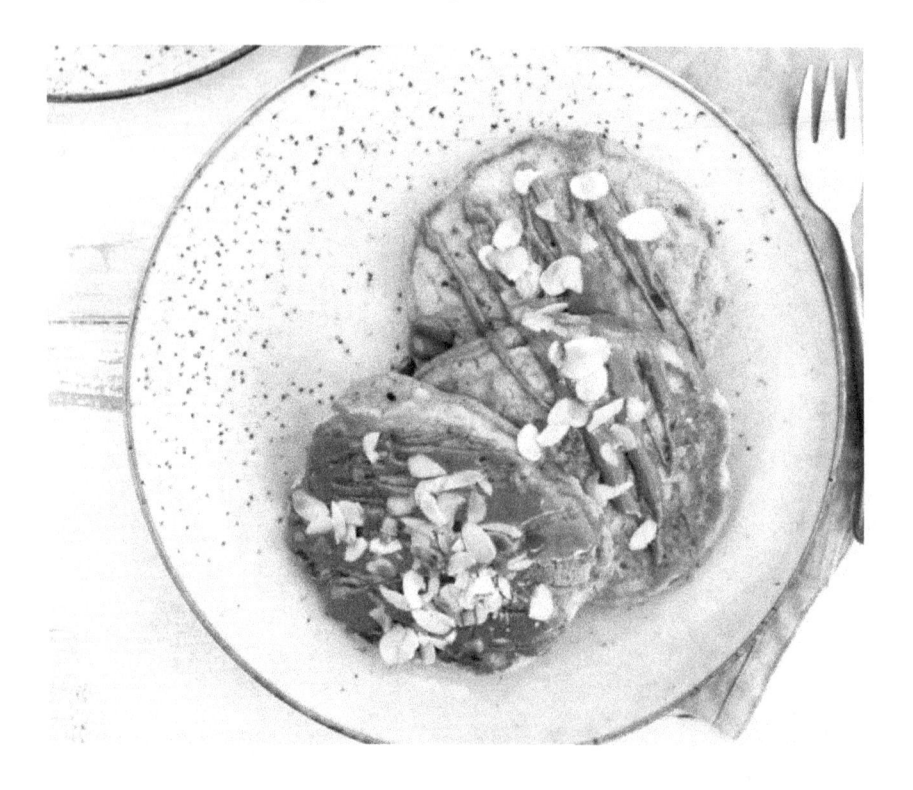

Ingredients:

- 1 cup almond flour
- ¾ cup tapioca flour
- 1 Tbsp. baking powder
- 2/3 teaspoon apple pie spice
- 1/3 cup unsweetened almond milk
- 2/3 teaspoon apple cider vinegar
- ½ tablespoon coconut oil, melted
- 1/3 tsp. pure vanilla extract

Directions:

Mix together almond flour, tapioca flour, baking powder, apple pie spice, unsweetened almond milk, apple cider vinegar, coconut oil, vanilla extract.

Pour a small amount on griddle, they will bubble around edges and throughout pancake, let cook 1 ½ - 2 minutes.

Amount per Serving:

- Calories 193
- % Daily Value*
- Total Fat 15.4g 20%
- Saturated Fat 2.5g 13%
- Cholesterol 0mg 0%
- Sodium 29mg 1%
- Total Carbohydrate 8.4g 3%
- Dietary Fiber 3.2g 11%
- Total Sugars 0.1g
- Protein 6.1g
- Vitamin D 0mcg 1%
- Calcium 189mg 15%
- Iron 0mg 2%
- Potassium 398mg 8%

Pegan Veggie Frittata

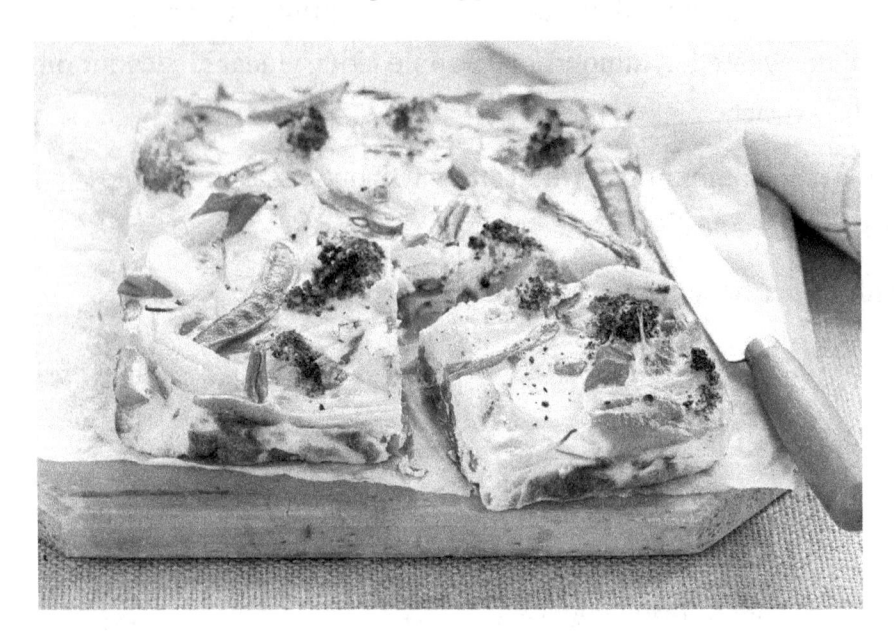

Great brunch treat!

Makes: 4-6 servings.

Ingredients:

- 6 eggs
- 1 Tbsp coconut oil
- 1/3 cup green olives, diced
- 1 red bell pepper, diced
- 2 shallots, thinly sliced
- 2 cups baby spinach
- Hot sauce or salsa

Directions:

In a large bowl mix together eggs, olives, bell pepper, shallots, baby spinach, hot sauce or salsa. Pour mixture into skillet and cook 5-8 minutes.

Store any leftovers in an airtight container and will keep 1 week.

Amount per Serving:

- Calories 113
- % Daily Value*
- Total Fat 8.2g 10%
- Saturated Fat 4g 20%
- Cholesterol 196mg 65%
- Sodium 93mg 4%
- Total Carbohydrate 3.4g 1%
- Dietary Fiber 0.6g 2%
- Total Sugars 1.7g
- Protein 7.3g
- Vitamin D 18mcg 92%
- Calcium 44mg 3%
- Iron 1mg 8%
- Potassium 196mg 4%

Eggs in Acorn Squash

Keep an eye out for seasonal melons!

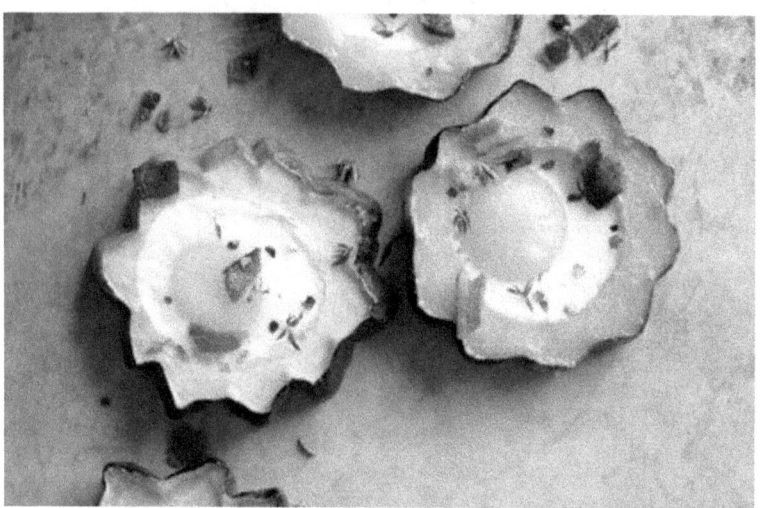

Makes: 2 servings.

Ingredients:

- 1 acorn squash
- ½ tsp smoked paprika
- ¼ tsp black pepper
- 2/3 teaspoon coconut extract
- 2 Tbsp olive oil
- 2 large eggs
- ¼ cup shredded Monterey jack
- 2 tablespoon chopped thyme

Directions:

Preheat oven to 425 and line a baking tray with parchment paper.

Cut 2-3 slits across squash and microwave 2 minutes. Cut off top and bottom then cut into two pieces; remove seeds and spoon out hole in middle.

Mix together smoked paprika, pepper, coconut extract, and olive oil. Brush on squash and bake 20-30 minutes.

Put an egg in hole and bake another 10-12 minutes.

Amount per Serving:

- Calories 282
- % Daily Value*
- Total Fat 17g 22%
- Saturated Fat 5.2g 26%
- Cholesterol 201mg 67%
- Sodium 168mg 7%
- Total Carbohydrate 25.6g 9%
- Dietary Fiber 4.5g 16%
- Total Sugars 0.5g
- Protein 11.9g
- Vitamin D 18mcg 88%
- Calcium 251mg 19%
- Iron 6mg 33%
- Potassium 852mg 18%

Collard & Tomato Omelet

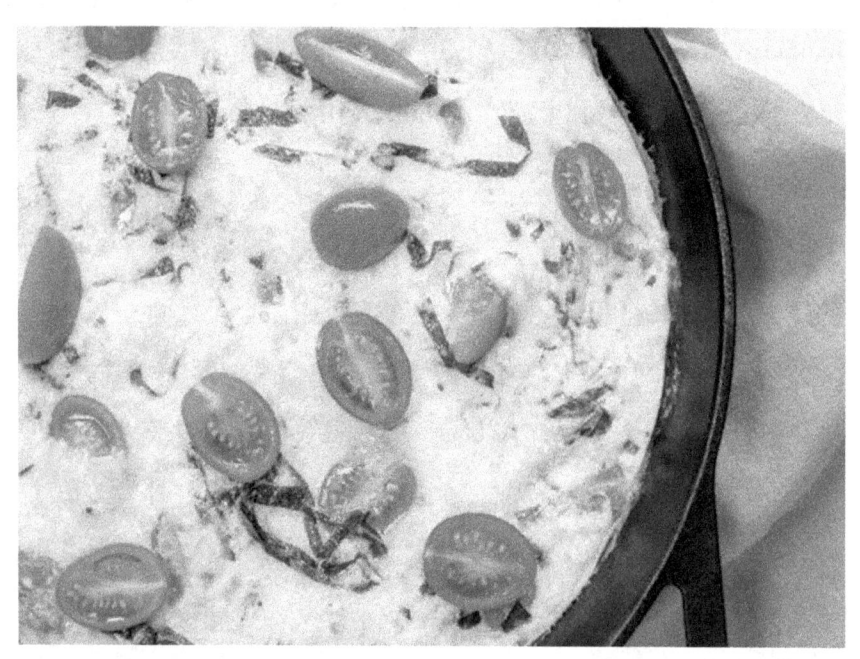

Spinach or kale works, too!

Makes: 1 serving.

Ingredients:

- 2 Tbsp unsalted butter, divided
- 3-4 cups collard greens
- 2 tablespoons chicken stock or water, more if needed
- 2 tablespoon chipotles peppers, diced
- ½ teaspoon turmeric (optional)
- 4 large eggs
- Chopped parsley or cilantro for top

Directions:

Over medium-high heat melt butter then cook pancetta 8-9 minutes; then, add collard greens, peppers, and stock/water.

In a small skillet, add 1 tablespoon of butter and let melt until emitting a nutty scent. Beat eggs and pour into skillet and cook 1 minute.

Flip right edge over and align with left side. Will be done when all of eggs liquid has cooked up.

Transfer to plate and spoon collards down the center.

Amount per Serving:

- *Calories 523*
- *% Daily Value**
- *Total Fat 42.7g 55%*
- *Saturated Fat 20.1g 101%*
- *Cholesterol 716mg 239%*
- *Sodium 768mg 33%*
- *Total Carbohydrate 12.7g 5%*
- *Dietary Fiber 6.7g 24%*
- *Total Sugars 3.5g*
- *Protein 25.6g*
- *Vitamin D 78mcg 388%*
- *Calcium 254mg 20%*
- *Iron 4mg 25%*

- *Potassium 272mg 6%*

Herbed Mushrooms, Avocado and Eggs in a Bell Pepper

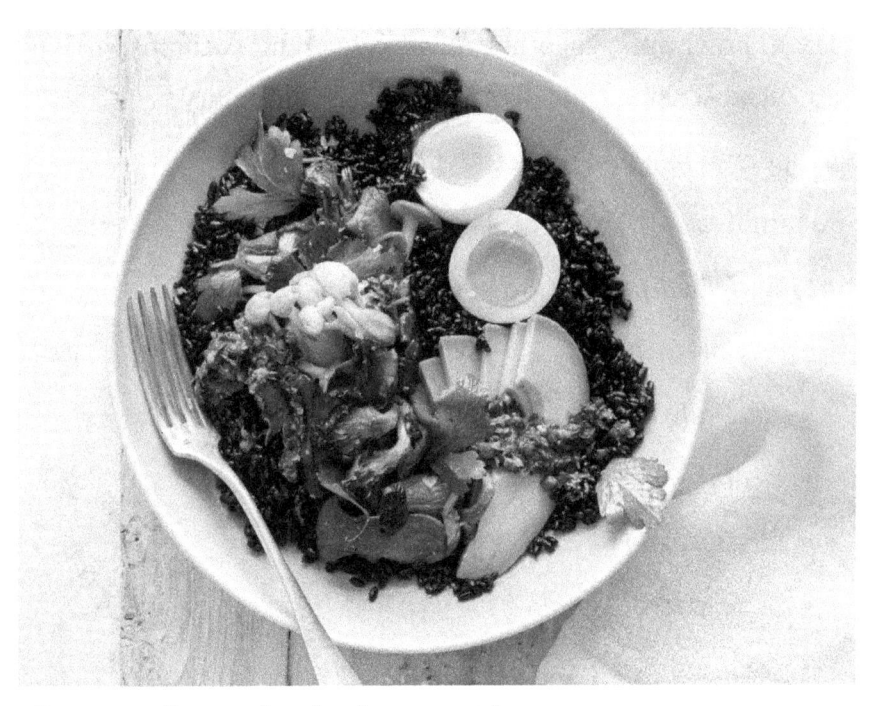

Great use for garden fresh peppers!

Makes: 2 servings.

Ingredients:

- 2 eggs
- 1/3 cup diced mushrooms
- 1/3 cup diced avocado
- ¼ cup scallions, diced
- 1 teaspoon oregano, diced
- 1 teaspoon rosemary, diced
- ¾ cup water or chicken stock

- 2 red bell peppers; seeds, stems, and ribs removed

Directions:

Preheat oven to 350 and prepare 9x9 dish.

In a large bowl mix together eggs, diced mushrooms, diced avocado, diced scallions, diced oregano, diced rosemary.

Place peppers in pan and fill both with mix.

Bake 30 minutes.

Amount per Serving:

- Calories 161
- % Daily Value*
- Total Fat 9.6g 12%
- Saturated Fat 2.4g 12%
- Cholesterol 164mg 55%
- Sodium 72mg 3%
- Total Carbohydrate 13.6g 5%
- Dietary Fiber 4.3g 15%
- Total Sugars 7g
- Protein 7.9g
- Vitamin D 57mcg 287%
- Calcium 67mg 5%
- Iron 3mg 14%
- Potassium 492mg 10%

AM Smoothie

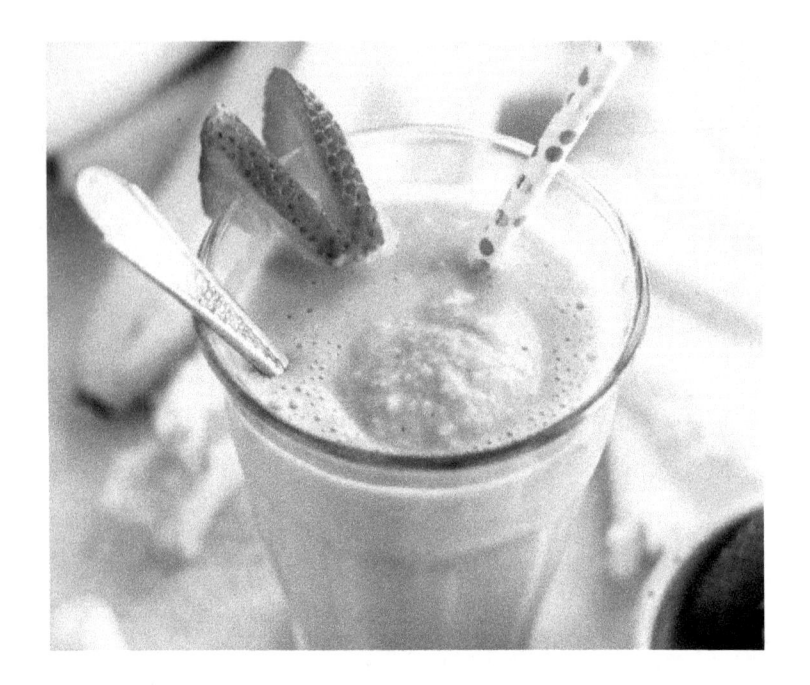

A great way to start the morning!

Makes: 1 serving.

Ingredients:

- ¾ cup coconut milk
- 1 chilled banana, sliced
- 1 ½ cups strawberries, heads chopped off
- 1 teaspoon mint flavored extract
- 1 cup ice

Directions:

Blend together coconut milk, sliced banana, beheaded strawberries, mint extract, ice.

Enjoy!

Amount per Serving:

- Calories 588
- % Daily Value*
- Total Fat 44g 56%
- Saturated Fat 38.2g 191%
- Cholesterol 0mg 0%
- Sodium 30mg 1%
- Total Carbohydrate 53.5g 19%
- Dietary Fiber 11.4g 41%
- Total Sugars 31g
- Protein 6.9g
- Vitamin D 0mcg 0%
- Calcium 69mg 5%
- Iron 4mg 23%
- Potassium 1226mg 26%

Easy Dairy-Free Latte

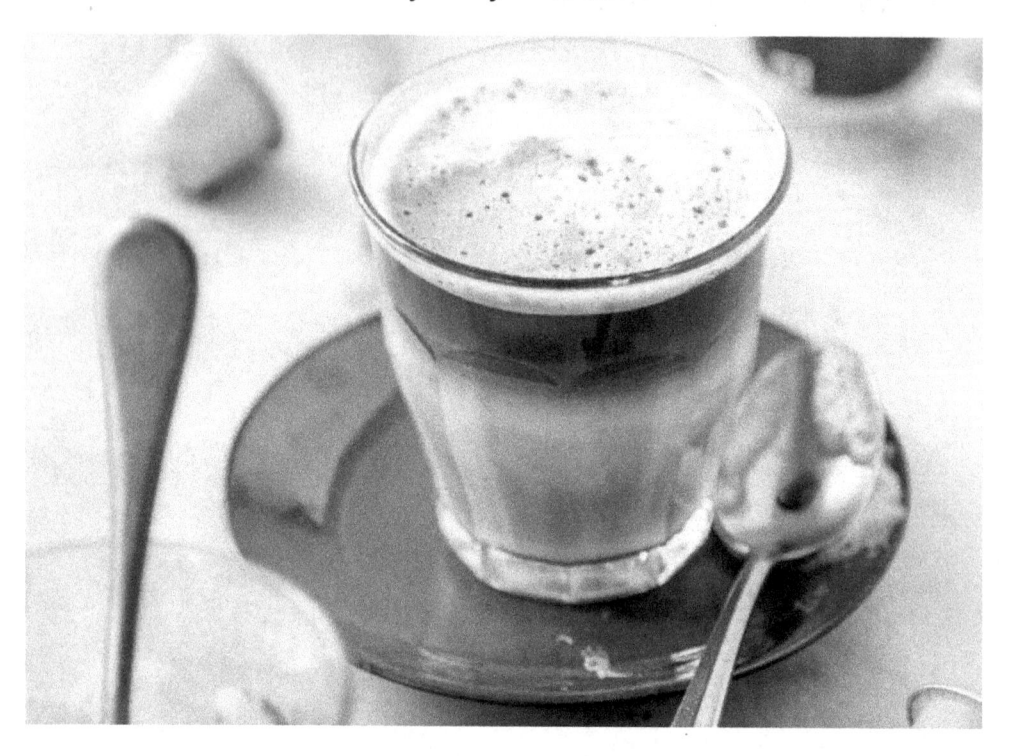

Great afternoon treat!

Makes: 1 serving.

Ingredients:

- 1 6 oz. serving strong coffee
- 3-4 tablespoons of cashews
- 2-3 teaspoons honey

Directions:

Blend coffee, cashews, and honey together starting low and working to high for about 40-45 seconds.

Amount per Serving:

- Calories 245
- % Daily Value*
- Total Fat 15.9g 20%
- Saturated Fat 3.2g 16%
- Cholesterol 0mg 0%
- Sodium 11mg 0%
- Total Carbohydrate 22.8g 8%
- Dietary Fiber 1.1g 4%
- Total Sugars 13.2g
- Protein 5.6g
- Vitamin D 0mcg 0%
- Calcium 16mg 1%
- Iron 2mg 12%
- Potassium 202mg 4%

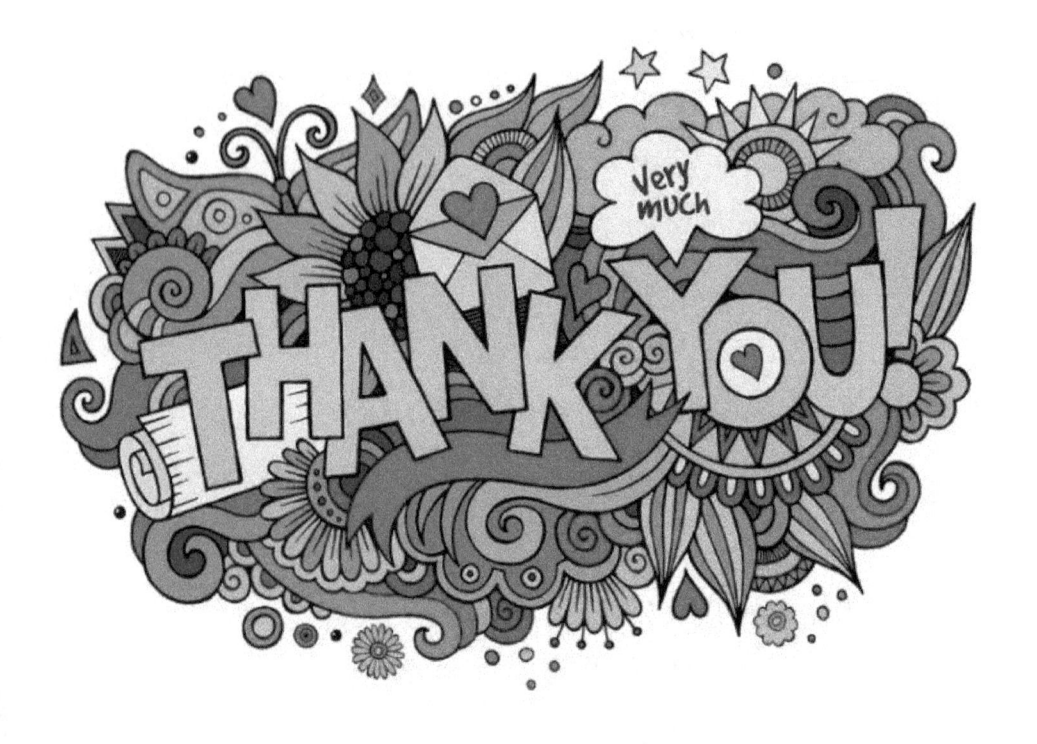

Author's Afterthoughts

Thanks ever so much to each of my cherished readers for investing the time to read this book!

I know you could have picked from many other books, but you chose this one. So, a big thanks for reading all the way to the end. If you enjoyed this book or received value from it, I'd like to ask you for a favor. Please take a few minutes to **post an honest and**

heartfelt review on *Amazon.com.* Your support does make a difference and helps to benefit other people.

Thanks!

D.Robert Marshall

About the Author

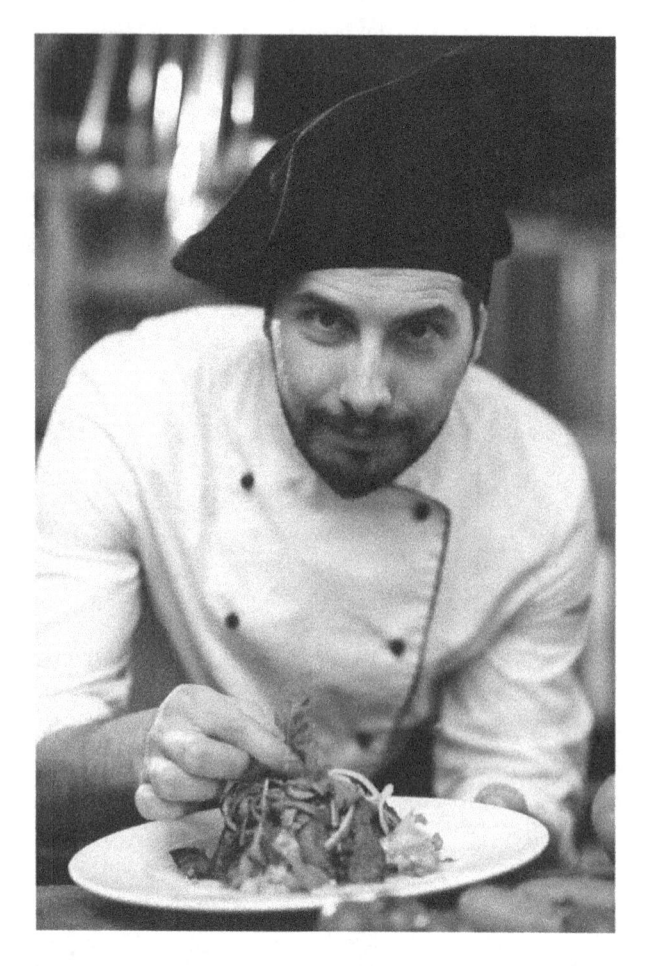

D.Robert Marshall

Robert received his culinary degree from Le Counte' School of Culinary Delights in Paris, France. He enjoyed cooking more than any of his former positions. Hi lived in Montgomery, Alabama most of his life. Hi married Roberta Capri and moved with her to Paris as he pursued his career in journalism. During the time he was there, he joined several cooking groups to learn the French cuisine, which inspired him to go to school and become a great chef.

Robert has achieved many awards in the field of food preparation. He has taught at several different culinary schools. He is in high demand on the talk show circulation, sharing her knowledge and recipes. Robert's favorite pastime is learning new ways to cook old dishes.

Robert is now writing cookbooks to add to her long list of achievements. The present one consists of favorite recipes as well as a few culinary delights from other cultures. He expands everyone's expectations on how to achieve wonderful dishes and not spend a lot of money. Robert firmly believes a wonderful dish can be prepare out of common household staples.

If anyone is interested in collecting Robert's cookbooks, check out your local bookstores and online. They are a big seller whatever venue you choose to purchase from.